Qualitative Research Methods in Mental Health and Psychotherapy

Qualitative Research Methods in Mental Health and Psychotherapy

A Guide for Students and Practitioners

Edited by David Harper and
Andrew R. Thompson

WILEY-BLACKWELL

A John Wiley & Sons, Ltd., Publication

Wiley-Blackwell is an imprint of John Wiley & Sons, formed by the merger of Wiley's global Scientific, Technical and Medical business with Blackwell Publishing.

Registered Office
John Wiley & Sons Ltd, The Atrium, Southern Gate, Chichester, West Sussex, PO19 8SQ, United Kingdom

Editorial Offices
350 Main Street, Malden, MA 02148-5020, USA
9600 Garsington Road, Oxford, OX4 2DQ, UK
The Atrium, Southern Gate, Chichester, West Sussex, PO19 8SQ, UK

For details of our global editorial offices, for customer services, and for information about how to apply for permission to reuse the copyright material in this book please see our website at www.wiley.com/wiley-blackwell.

Library of Congress Cataloging-in-Publication Data

Qualitative research methods in mental health and psychotherapy : a guide for students and practitioners / edited by David Harper & Andrew R. Thompson.
     p. ; cm.
  Includes bibliographical references and index.
   ISBN 978-0-470-66373-8 (cloth) – ISBN 978-0-470-66370-7 (pbk.)
  1. Mental health.   2. Qualitative research.   3. Psychotherapy–Methodology.   I. Harper, David, 1965–   II. Thompson, Andrew R. (Andrew Robert), 1970–
   [DNLM: 1. Mental Disorders.   2. Qualitative Research.   3. Psychotherapy–methods.   WM 20]
   RA790.Q34 2012
   616.89–dc22   2010052118

A catalogue record for this book is available from the British Library.

This book is published in the following electronic formats: ePDFs 9781119973256; Wiley Online Library 9781119973249

Typeset in 10.5/13pt Minion by Aptara Inc., New Delhi, India

1   2012

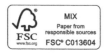

Contents

About the Contributors

Evrinomy Avdi is a clinical psychologist and Senior Lecturer in Clinical Psychology at the School of Psychology of the Aristotle University of Thessaloniki, Greece. Her research interests lie in the application of discourse and narrative analytic approaches to the study of various domains of clinical psychology practice, and more specifically diagnosis, psychotherapy and the experience of living with cancer. She is interested in exploring the links between deconstructive research and actual clinical practice.

Abi Billin completed her counselling psychology training at City University London in 2009 and was awarded a Doctorate in Counselling Psychology in 2010. She conducted her doctoral research into the experience of the end of life. Abi is interested in existential phenomenology and humanistic approaches to counselling psychology.

Eleni Chambers works as a researcher within the School of Health and Related Research at the University of Sheffield. Her background is in conflict resolution and mental health in a variety of settings, mainly in the voluntary sector. Eleni is also a long-term user of mental health services and brings this perspective to all her work. Her current interests are in user involvement in health and social care services and research, psychological therapies and self-management.

Kathy Charmaz is Professor of Sociology and Director of the Faculty Writing Program at Sonoma State University, a program for supporting faculty members' scholarly writing. She has written, co-authored or co-edited nine books including *Constructing Grounded Theory: A Practical Guide through Qualitative Analysis*, which has been translated into Chinese, Japanese, Polish and Portuguese. Among her most recent writings are two multi-authored books, *Five Ways of Doing Qualitative Analysis: Phenomenological Psychology, Grounded Theory, Discourse Analysis, Narrative Research, and Intuitive Inquiry*, forthcoming with Guilford and *Developing Grounded Theory: The Second Generation*. She is past-president of the Society for the Study of Symbolic Interaction.

Phillip Dyson is a graduate student in the Faculty of Health and Social Care at the Open University. His research explores the different ways used to explain and make sense of 'what is going on' in self-harm. He is pursuing this through three identities – researcher as 'voyeur' (scrutinizing Facebook postings); researcher as 'lurker' (listening in on conversations going on in online chatrooms); and researcher as 'detective' (using Q methodology). He is particularly interested in discovering how innovations in IT can open up new methodological frontiers, boldly going to places never reached before.

Robert Elliott , is Professor of Counselling in the Counselling Unit at the University of Strathclyde. A Professor Emeritus of Psychology at the University of Toledo (Ohio), he is co-author of four books, including *Learning Process-Experiential Psychotherapy* (2004), and *Research Methods in Clinical Psychology* (2002), as well as more than 120 journal articles and book chapters. He previously co-edited *Psychotherapy Research* and *Person-Centered Counseling and Psychotherapies*. In 2008 he received both the Distinguished Research Career Award of the Society for Psychotherapy Research, and the Carl Rogers Award from the Division of Humanistic Psychology of the American Psychological Association.

Alison Faulkner is a freelance researcher, trainer and consultant, working from a service user perspective. She has over 20 years' experience of social research mainly in the mental health field, and has worked for most of the national mental health charities. Alison is herself a mental health service user/survivor, and has written and presented extensively on the subject. In a freelance capacity, she drafted the guidance on service user involvement for the MHRN Service User Research Group, England, and researched and wrote *The Ethics of Survivor Research* for the Joseph Rowntree Foundation (Policy Press, 2004). She was a co-editor of *This is Survivor Research* (PCCS Books, 2009).

Hannah Frith is a Senior Lecturer in Psychology at the University of Brighton. Her research interests cover visual identity, body image, sexuality and mental health. Underpinning these varied interests is a focus on embodiment and exploring ways in which being in the body is socially constructed. Hannah uses a range of qualitative methods to explore these issues and recently her research has explored the use of visual methods to explore embodied experience (such as the experience of undergoing chemotherapy). She has become interested in analysing media texts which present multi-faceted representations of embodiment such as 'How to Look Good Naked'.

Eugenie Georgaca is Senior Lecturer in Clinical Psychology at the School of Psychology of the Aristotle University of Thessaloniki, Greece. She teaches, researches and publishes in the area of clinical psychology, psychotherapy and mental health, and especially qualitative methodology, psychoanalysis and critical perspectives on psychopathology. She was a co-author of *Deconstructing Psychopathology* (Sage, 1995) and has published articles on psychotic discourse, delusions, discursive approaches to analysing psychotherapy, discourse analysis and social constructionist notions of subjectivity.

Kate Gleeson is an independent trainer in research and professional development. This follows a 25 year career in higher education which culminated in 7 years as Research Director on the Bristol Doctorate in Clinical Psychology. Kate's research interests lie in visual identity and personhood, and in developing research methods that enable an exploration of visuality and subjectivity. Kate's most recent projects have focused on the visual identity of young women and people with learning disabilities.

David Harper is Reader in Clinical Psychology at the University of East London (UEL). His research interests are in critical psychology and social constructionist approaches in mental health, particularly in relation to psychosis. He is a co-author of *Deconstructing Psychopathology* (Sage, 1995) and a member of UEL's Psychology and Social Change research group. He works one session a week as a Consultant Clinical Psychologist for East London NHS Foundation Trust.

Helene Joffe is a Reader in Social and Health Psychology in the Division of Psychology and Language Sciences, University College London (UCL). Her area of interest is public engagement with risks ranging from emerging infectious diseases to earthquakes and climate change. She uses thematic analysis in studying these phenomena and teaches this method at a post-graduate level at UCL.

Michael Larkin works as a Senior Lecturer in Psychology on the University of Birmingham's doctoral training course for Clinical Psychology. He has a specific interest in phenomenological and cultural approaches to psychology. Much of his research explores the experiences of families and young people who are using psychology services.

Michael Murray is Professor of Social and Health Psychology at Keele University, UK. Prior to that, he held appointments at other universities in England, Northern Ireland and Canada. He has (co-)edited several collections on critical and qualitative approaches to health psychology including *Qualitative Health Psychology: Theories and Methods* (with Chamberlain, Sage 1999) and *Critical Health Psychology* (Palgrave, 2004). He has also published articles and chapters on narrative psychology in the *Journal of Health Psychology*, *Social Science Information* and in several edited collections. His current research interests include the use of participatory methods to engage communities in various forms of collective action.

Mark Rapley is Professor of Clinical Psychology at the University of East London. He is the author of *The Social Construction of Intellectual Disability* (Cambridge University Press), *Quality of Life Research* (Sage) and, with Susan Hansen and Alec McHoul, *Beyond Help* (PCCS Books). He lives in London, but wishes he did not.

Sally Sargeant is a Lecturer in Psychology at Keele University and a chartered member of the British Psychological Society. She has diverse interests that span chronic illness, mental health, consumer behaviour and the psychology of art. Her PhD work developed an audio diary intervention for young people with a chronic illness, which led to her interest in qualitative health research. Sally's more recent projects involve examining children's levels of trust in their physicians, and also psychological implications of new breast cancer treatment pathways.

Rachel Shaw is a Health Psychologist registered with the Health Professions Council and a Chartered Psychologist of the British Psychological Society (BPS). She is Honorary Secretary of the Qualitative Methods in Psychology Section of the BPS. Rachel currently works as a Lecturer in the School of Life and Health Sciences at Aston University. Her research interests include illness experience, health management, media framing of health issues, meta-synthesis of qualitative evidence, interpretative phenomenology and reflexivity. Rachel has publications in health psychology and qualitative methodology in psychology. She is also author of several chapters in qualitative methods textbooks.

Liz Spencer is a research consultant with more than 30 years' experience of qualitative methods in both academic and applied policy research. She is currently a Research Associate at the University of Essex, as well as an academician of the Academy of Social Sciences (AcSS).

Jane Ritchie was the founder and first Director of the Qualitative Research Unit at the National Centre for Social Research and is an AcSS. With Liz Spencer, whilst at NatCen, she conducted a review of quality in qualitative research and evaluation for the UK Cabinet Office, which is widely respected and used by researchers.

Wendy Stainton Rogers is Professor of Health Psychology at the Open University and is an internationally recognized expert in Q methodology. Her publications include *Explaining Health and Illness* (1991) and *The Psychology of Gender and Sexuality* (2001) (with the late Rex Stainton Rogers). In 2009, she co-edited (with Carla Willig) *The Sage Handbook of Qualitative Research in Psychology* and is currently producing a second edition of her *Social Psychology: Experimental and Critical Approaches*, to be published in 2011. She was a member of the NICE Development Group on Behaviour Change, and is currently the Chair of the International Society for Critical Health Psychology (ISCHP).

Andrew Thompson is a Reader in Clinical Psychology. He is a Chartered Clinical and Health Psychologist. He is the Director of Research Training at the Clinical Psychology Unit at the University of Sheffield. He is clinically active and is also a practitioner of cognitive analytic therapy. He has a long-standing interest in the use of qualitative methods in clinical psychology and has supervised many mental health practitioners and trainee clinical psychologists in the use of such methods. His research interests focus on adjustment to appearance altering conditions.

Alison Tweed is Clinical Director and Principal Lecturer on the Doctoral Clinical Psychology Training Programme based at the Universities of Staffordshire and Keele. She is a clinical psychologist and qualitative researcher with interests in the areas of medical psychology, particularly chronic illness and clinical psychology training. Her current research involves the evaluation of new innovations in the assessment of trainees' therapeutic skills within a competency-based framework.

Carla Willig is Professor of Psychology at City University London. She is also a counselling psychologist with an interest in existential phenomenological approaches to psychotherapy and counselling. Carla has a long-standing interest in qualitative research methodology and she has published books and papers concerned with both methodological and epistemological issues. Recently, Carla has begun to bring together her interests in counselling and qualitative research by exploring the meaning and practice of 'interpretation'.

Acknowledgements

David Harper would like to thank Sarah Amoss, Gary Brown, Pippa Dell, Ken Gannon, Mick McKeown, Ian Parker, Neil Rees, Sam Warner and Carla Willig for helpful exchanges about various aspects of the book. In addition, I owe a debt of gratitude to the University of East London's Psychology and Social Change research group, the clinical psychology programme team and past and present trainees and research supervisees. Many thanks to Andrew for having the initial idea, inviting me to join him and for his hard work and support over the last 2 years.

Andrew Thompson would like to thank the University of Sheffield for its generosity in granting a period of study leave which allowed the transformation of the idea for this book to make it into a proposal. A particularly big thank you to David for joining me in this venture and making it a reality.

Thanks are due to Wiley-Blackwell for their support with the project. Lastly, we both want to express our gratitude to the contributors who have been unfailingly generous in responding to our editorial requests. All research participants' identifying details have been anonymized.

Part I

Getting Started

Part I

Getting Started

1

Introduction

Andrew R. Thompson and David Harper

This book aims to provide a user-friendly introduction to the qualitative methods most commonly used in the mental health and psychotherapy arenas. A number of different professional groups and academic disciplines contribute to mental health care and our aim in putting together this book has been to create a text that shows how qualitative methods can generate knowledge specifically relevant to mental health and also to show how these approaches have the potential to improve practice and drive policy. We envisage this book being read by students, trainees and qualified practitioners from a variety of professions: clinical psychology; mental health nursing; social work; psychiatry; occupational therapy; family therapy; and those working in a wide variety of psychological therapies.

Mental health practitioners are used to working alongside their clients or with service users (we shall use these terms interchangeably throughout), with the aim of enhancing emotional well-being. Most will be trained to understand the phenomenon of mental distress from an individualized or *idiographic* perspective that acknowledges the role of social and cultural as well as biological influences upon behaviour, affect and experience. As such they will be used to '*collecting data*' and '*making sense of*' peoples' complex and rich personal histories and experiences in order to deliver care and support. Indeed, as we discuss below, several therapeutic approaches have their origins in qualitative and subjective exploration.

Although caution should be expressed in naively assuming counselling and other practitioner competencies can be simply transferred into the research setting (see Thompson & Russo, in press), we believe that many of the core competencies of mental health practitioners are highly transferable. However, for many the transfer of these competencies somehow gets lost when they move between practitioner and researcher roles. Consequently, it is our core ambition with this book to help both student and

Qualitative Research Methods in Mental Health and Psychotherapy: A Guide for Students and Practitioners, First Edition.
Edited by D. Harper and A.R. Thompson.

qualified mental health practitioner understand qualitative approaches, so as to have the confidence to conduct creative qualitative research of a high standard.

In order to achieve this aim we asked all of our contributors to describe their particular approach with reference to practical examples and to be clear about the sorts of questions the approach was most suited to address. We also asked them to clarify the philosophical underpinnings associated with the approach – an aspect of qualitative research, which often appears mystifying but is essential to get to grips with. As such we were explicit in our desire for contributors to detail the *epistemological tradition* of the approach covered. Epistemology is essentially the philosophical theory of knowledge, which addresses questions about how we can know what we know, and whether this knowledge is reliable or not. It is important to clarify how a method is positioned in relation to these questions in order to make sense of the findings.

Finally, we have encouraged our contributors to consider how qualitative researchers can more actively engage service users and the wider public. There has been a major policy push within mental health practice, policy and research to be inclusive of service users. Indeed, ethics committees explicitly request information on how service users have been consulted in relation to all aspects of proposed research. Service user researchers are making an increasing contribution to mental health research. Active involvement of service users at all levels of research from commissioning, collaboration and acting as lead researchers is likely to widen the types of questions asked by qualitative researchers (both from practitioner and service user backgrounds). Each chapter of this book has a section dedicated to considering the involvement of service users and participants and, in addition, there is a chapter focused specifically on service user involvement in research (see Chapter 4).

A Short and a Long History of the Use of Qualitative Methods in Mental Health Practice

Whilst qualitative research has a long history in disciplines like anthropology, it has only recently become more popular in disciplines like psychology allied to mental health. Having said this, significant psychotherapeutic approaches such as psychoanalysis and the humanistic therapies have their roots in detailed idiographic case studies (Ponterotto *et al.*, 2008).

Within our own discipline of psychology, the 1970s and 1980s saw heated methodological debates about the dominance of quantitative research in psychology and the reliance on laboratory experiments and questionnaires. Debates concerned ecological validity, the importance of language and context and so on. At this time many qualitative articles included a critique of quantitative methods to support the rationale for a qualitative study. However, over time, acceptance has grown and, since the 1990s, qualitative methods have achieved disciplinary legitimization in the United Kingdom (Henwood *et al.*, 1998). Qualitative methods are now routinely covered in most research methods textbooks in mental health and psychotherapy (often alongside quantitative methods), international and national journals have published qualitative studies and there are indications of the growing popularity of qualitative methods amongst some groups of trainee mental health professionals (e.g., Harper, in press). However, there is still some prejudice (and misunderstanding) – for example, many academic journals aimed at mental health practitioners still publish few if any qualitative studies and reviewers often return manuscripts with comments about sample size or reliability that are simply not appropriate (Harper, 2008).

As Willig and Stainton-Rogers (2008) have stated in their handbook of qualitative research in psychology 'there should be no more need to justify the use of qualitative methods than there is to justify quantitative methods' (p. 5) and this is a position we strongly concur with. At the same time, there is a need for an improvement in the quality of qualitative research and we believe this is best achieved by greater attention being paid to epistemological issues rather than to method per se (see Curt, 1994, on methodolatry).

What Can Qualitative Research Do?

There are many different qualitative methodologies, and all of them share an interest in detailed readings of qualitative material and understanding process rather than establishing causal relationships or quantifying the size or extent of something. Clearly, qualitative research will not help address questions that are primarily quantitative – for example, identifying the prevalence of a particular condition. However, the following questions are only really answerable with qualitative methodologies:

- What is it like to receive a diagnosis of personality disorder?
- How do therapists address ruptures in therapy?
- How do mental health practitioners communicate complex information?
- How do therapists contribute to service users' views of themselves?
- What is it like to receive cognitive analytic therapy?
- What are mental health nurses' experience of working with people who engage in self-harm?
- How are mental health problems constructed in the media?

Qualitative approaches enable *understanding of experience and processes.* Clearly, answering such questions is of importance in developing an understanding of emotional distress and increasing the quality of mental health practice. Thankfully, over recent years there has been an increased emphasis on quality and outcome rather than purely upon the numbers of people receiving a service. This has led to calls for qualitative research expertise (e.g., the White Paper: Equity and Excellence – Liberating the NHS; http://tinyurl.com/2a8ljeo). Of course, one of the contributions that qualitative research can make to policy debates is to help rethink the assumptive framework on which policy is based. Some research, like Boyle's (1997) work on abortion, reconceptualizes policy questions, interrogates the underlying assumptions that shape those questions and delineates normative discourses, reporting alternative or marginalized discourses. Indeed, alternative epistemological frameworks like social constructionism and critical realism can be useful political interventions in and of themselves (Shakespeare, 1998).

Types of Qualitative Research and the Importance of Reflexivity

A simple (but nonetheless helpful) distinction has been made between '*big q*' and '*little q*' methods (Kidder & Fine, 1987, 1997; see also Rowan, 2006; Willig, 2001). Research defined as little q broadly focuses on qualitative methods of data *collection*, usually from within a *realist* framework where there is an assumed direct relationship between what is observed and the nature of reality, where the researcher 'decides on the questions and processes the results in an objective fashion, keeping control of all aspects of the work' (Rowan, 2006, p. 16). Types of methods that might sometimes be described as little q include structured analyses of open responses to questionnaire questions, observer ratings of structured or semi-structured interviews and so on. Here, the aim will be to objectively capture, either to describe or to examine the extent to which data fit a particular framework. 'Big q' research (the focus of this book) is quite different, and is concerned with qualitative methods of *analysis* – that is, collecting and engaging with data in a more reflexive fashion, acknowledging (and using) the *intersubjective relationship* between the researcher and the researched (for a thorough introduction to these issues see Finlay & Gough, 2003). As such, big q research involves careful consideration of *reflexivity*. This is a slippery concept in its own right, which has been used (and misused) to mean a variety of things but generally refers to the ability to engage critically in understanding the contribution the researcher's experiences and circumstances have had in shaping a given study (and its findings). This is sometimes separated out into two strands: *epistemological reflexivity* and *personal reflexivity*. Personal reflexivity concerns the influences of the researcher's own history, whereas epistemological reflexivity concerns exploring how the assumptions of the approach taken shaped the study. Again we can see the crucial importance of being able to stand back from one's study and oneself, so as to consider how the approach one has taken answers questions about how, and what, we can know (Willig, 2001).

This split between different types of qualitative methods is grossly simplistic and numerous writers have produced complex frameworks to account for the epistemological positions of different approaches, which is discussed in more detail in Chapter 7.

What is in the Book

The book has three sections, beginning with a section on *getting started*. The second section is dedicated to *different methods* and all of the chapters contain helpful further reading resources and also include examples of studies and of the analysis process itself. The third section is a concluding section, including a chapter on *establishing quality* in qualitative research in mental health, and our concluding chapter, discussing our views on emerging themes and future developments in qualitative research. We consider the first and third sections to be essential reading at least for those new to qualitative research and we would deter readers from just focusing on the chapter that covers the method they are currently planning on using.

The skills required to undertake a literature review are often underestimated and Rachel Shaw in Chapter 2 describes in detail how to identify and synthesize qualitative literature. In Chapter 3, Andrew Thompson and Eleni Chambers describe some of the unique ethical dilemmas that need to be considered when conducting qualitative research. In Chapter 4, Alison Faulkner describes the history of service user involvement in mental health research and sets out principles and resources so as to enable collaborative research between practitioners and service users. Data collection is often not given enough attention in the planning of qualitative research, and in Chapters 5 (Hannah Frith and Kate Gleeson) and 6 (Robert Elliott), some of the key issues that need to be considered in the choice of data collection techniques are discussed. Chapter 6 specifically focuses on collecting data in the context of exploring psychotherapy change processes; this chapter covers a range of methodologies and was included in this section because it demonstrates the unique tradition that qualitative research has developed for exploring and collecting data in relation to psychotherapy process. In the last chapter in this section, David Harper examines the epistemological assumptions of the different research traditions and discusses how one might choose between different methods.

Part II focuses on a range of methods. It is a wide but not exhaustive grouping. Each chapter contains practical information as to how to go about conducting a study within the approach. In order for the book to be easy to navigate we asked the authors of these chapters to address key questions. As such each chapter includes a description of the method and its history. Key epistemological assumptions are considered as are the kind of research questions the method is most suited to addressing and what kind of data are appropriate. The involvement of service users and participants is explicitly considered. Each chapter includes a step-by-step guide to how to use the method including a worked example. Contributors then identify if there are any particular issues to be considered when evaluating the quality of a study using this method. Finally, each chapter concludes with a discussion of how the method can influence policy and practice and if there are any recent innovations in the use of the method. This consistency also aids comparison between methods.

In Part III, in Chapter 16, Liz Spencer and Jane Ritchie deal with evaluating the quality of qualitative research. The danger is that, as many of us discover, inappropriate quality criteria can be applied by supervisors, examiners and reviewers. Unfortunately, some widely cited criteria for evaluating qualitative research are appropriate only for evaluating more realist or phenomenological research. The more inclusive approach advocated in Chapter 16 seems a potentially more useful approach and we hope it gains wider currency within mental health research.

We hope that the book will not only be practically useful, but also inspiring – encouraging the development of rigorous and collaborative research that will make a difference to mental health theory, policy, and practice.

References

Boyle, M. (1997). *Re-thinking abortion: Psychology, gender, power and the law*. London: Routledge.

Curt, B. (1994). *Textuality and tectonics: Troubling social and psychological science*. Buckingham: Open University Press.

Finlay, L. & Gough, B. (Eds.) (2003). *Reflexivity: A practical guide for researchers in health and social sciences*. Oxford: Blackwell.

Guba, E.G. & Lincoln, Y.S. (1994). Competing paradigms in qualitative research. In N.K. Denzin & Y.S. Lincoln (Eds.) *Handbook of qualitative research* (pp. 105–117). Thousand Oaks, CA: Sage.

Harper, D. (2008). Clinical psychology. In C. Willig & W. Stainton-Rogers (Eds.) *The Sage handbook of qualitative research in psychology* (pp. 430–454). London: Sage.

Henwood, K., McQueen, C. & Vetere, A. (1998). Qualitative research and clinical psychology: Promoting the interchange. *Clinical Psychology Forum, 114*, 4–35.

Kidder, L.H. & Fine, M. (1987). Qualitative and quantitative methods: When stories converge. In M.M. Mark & L. Shotland (Eds.) *New directions in program evaluation* (pp. 57–75). San Francisco, CA: Jossey-Bass.

Kidder, L.H. & Fine, M. (1997). Qualitative inquiry in psychology: A radical tradition. In D. Fox & I. Prilleltensky (Eds.) *Critical psychology: An introduction* (pp. 34–50). London: Sage.

Ponterotto, J.G., Kuriakose, G. & Granovskaya, Y. (2008). Counselling and psychotherapy. In C. Willig & W. Stainton-Rogers (Eds.) *The Sage handbook of qualitative research in psychology* (pp. 1–12). London: Sage.

Rowan, J. (2006). An overview of qualitative methods in psychological research. *QMiP Newsletter, 1*, 16–17. Leicester: British Psychological Society.

Shakespeare, T. (1998). Social constructionism as a political strategy. In I. Velody & R. Williams (Eds.) *The politics of constructionism* (pp. 168–181). London: Sage.

Thompson, A.R. & Russo, K. (in press). Ethical dilemmas for clinical psychologists in conducting qualitative research. *Qualitative Research in Psychology*.

Willig, C. (2001). *Introducing qualitative research in psychology: Adventures in theory and method*. Buckingham: Open University Press.

Willig, C. (in press). Perspectives on the epistemological bases for qualitative research. In H. Cooper (Ed.) *The handbook of research methods in psychology*. Washington, DC: American Psychological Association.

Willig, C. & Stainton-Rogers, W. (2008). Introduction. In C. Willig & W. Stainton-Rogers (Eds.) *The Sage handbook of qualitative research in psychology* (pp. 1–12). London: Sage.

2

Identifying and Synthesizing Qualitative Literature

Rachel L. Shaw

The ability to locate, review and synthesize literature are essential competencies required by mental health practitioners, students and trainees in order for not only formation of new research proposals, but also continuing professional development. This chapter will do two things: (i) provide instruction on conducting a systematic literature review that includes qualitative research; and (ii) outline and illustrate one way of carrying out a meta-synthesis of qualitative evidence.

Fitting Qualitative Research into the Hierarchy of Evidence

The growth and significance of evidence-based practice within mental health and psychotherapy is clearly illustrated by the guidance from the National Institute for Health and Clinical Excellence (NICE, 2008) for the adoption of Cognitive Behavioural Therapy for the management of common mental health problems and the focus on developing and remaining faithful to guidelines for professional practice within specific interventions and methods of care as emphasized in the Increasing Access to Psychological Therapies Programme (IAPT: Department of Health, 2008). For practice to be informed by contemporary research evidence there is a requirement that such evidence is systematically reviewed and appraised in terms of its quality and effectiveness.

In the 1990s, the Cochrane Collaboration was established in the United Kingdom to fulfil that function; Cochrane reviews and updates interventions which have been tested in randomized control trials (RCTs). Indeed, it was Cochrane that helped to establish the systematic review of RCTs as the 'gold standard' for determining evidence-based practice (Guyatt *et al.*, 2000; Marks & Sykes, 2004). Nevertheless, any review of the literature

Qualitative Research Methods in Mental Health and Psychotherapy: A Guide for Students and Practitioners, First Edition.
Edited by D. Harper and A.R. Thompson.
© 2012 John Wiley & Sons, Ltd. Published 2012 by John Wiley & Sons, Ltd.

will illustrate that there are many other forms of evidence available that contribute to the knowledge base and that we should therefore also include in our reviews. The majority of research of relevance to mental health practitioners involves measuring clients' behaviour and mental state using standardized measures such as the Patient Health Questionnaire (PHQ9: Kroenke & Spitzer, 2002) and, more recently, there has been a significant increase in the amount of research employing qualitative methods particularly to explore issues in relation to psychotherapy process (see Chapter 6) such as *how* therapies or interventions might work (Elliott *et al.*, 1999).

Incorporating this variety of evidence into systematic reviews has been problematic but methods for including non-trial quantitative data in systematic reviews have been developed (Mulrow *et al.*, 1997). More challenging was the growing need to find ways of incorporating qualitative research into such reviews but, before that was possible, there first had to be a convincing argument that qualitative research was a credible source of evidence (Dixon-Woods *et al.*, 2001). The guidelines published by the NHS Centre for Reviews and Dissemination in 2001 went some way to establishing qualitative research as a valid and necessary source of evidence. Since then, the Cochrane Qualitative Research Methods Group (CQRMG) has been established to support the inclusion of qualitative evidence in systematic reviews and we have seen a phenomenal expansion in the use of qualitative research methods in clinical psychology, psychotherapy and mental health practice more generally (e.g., Golsworthy & Coyle, 2001; Larkin *et al.*, 2009; Martindale *et al.*, 2009; Midgley *et al.*, 2006;). This is encouraging and a further indicator of the need to establish methods for identifying this important evidence base and for the synthesis of qualitative research findings.

Identifying Qualitative Literature

In this section some generic tips for conducting a literature review are outlined before describing in more detail ways of identifying qualitative evidence.

Designing a search strategy

The key goal of any literature review is to be as comprehensive as possible and to en-sure reports retrieved (which may be journal articles but also 'grey literature' such as government reports, policy documents, professional guidelines and documents pub-lished by charities and non-governmental organizations) are relevant to the research or practice question posed. If the literature review is to form the basis for a systematic review, the search strategy must demonstrate comprehensiveness and be reproducible (NHS Centre for Reviews and Dissemination, 2001). Before embarking on a review of the evidence it is worth checking facilities such as the Cochrane Library to determine whether a search strategy related to your question has already been developed. Often it is acceptable to re-use published search strategies as there is no sense in re-inventing the wheel, although in some cases you may wish to scrutinize them carefully for in-appropriate or problematic assumptions or for omitted terms which may have been

Table 2.1   CHIP Tool

Study components	Description
Context	Early Intervention Service for Psychosis
How	Qualitative methods
Issues	Content/activities involved in the Service
	Accessibility of the Service
	Cultural/religious sensitivity of the Service
Population	Young South Asian men

introduced since the strategy was developed. If no such strategy exists, then it will be necessary to design a new one.

The first task is to develop a research question – the more focused it is, the better. Let us use the example of a project exploring young South Asian men's experiences of an Early Intervention Service for psychosis. An appropriate research question would be something as simple as: What are young South Asian men's experiences of an Early Intervention Service? The second task is to break down this question into its component parts. To help with this process, you may wish to use the CHIP Tool (Table 2.1; Shaw, 2010), which was designed for this purpose.

Now that the constituent parts of the research question are clear it can be helpful to develop a mind-map of all relevant keywords and synonyms you can think of. The terms identified during this activity will form the basis of your search strategy. Designing a search strategy is an iterative process (in so far as it will need revisiting as the search progresses). It is not always obvious which terms will be most successful in light of comprehensiveness and identification of relevant articles. The effectiveness of search strategies can be judged in terms of their powers for *recall* and *precision* (O'Rourke *et al.*, 1999; Diagnostic Strategies for Information Retrieval, 2004). These terms can be understood by drawing the analogy of a screening test: *recall* is likened to sensitivity (i.e., a strategy's ability to identify potentially relevant studies, those that 'tested positive'); *precision* indicates a strategy's ability to identify 'true positives' (i.e., articles recognized by the search terms that are relevant to your research question, 'diagnosed positive'). In designing your search strategy it is necessary to find a balance between these two criteria; clearly, a high recall, high precision strategy would be ideal but trade-offs between recall and precision are unavoidable (Buckland & Gey, 1994).

The best way of conducting a thorough and systematic literature search is through searching online bibliographical databases, such as MEDLINE and Web of Knowledge. Bibliographical databases are made up of indices of peer-reviewed journals and all articles published in those journals that are indexed are retrievable. One of the most extensive databases is Web of Knowledge, which includes science and social science journals as well as all journals indexed in MEDLINE, therefore extending its coverage to include medical literature. Other more specific databases exist, such as PsychInfo and CINAHL (Cumulative Index to Nursing and Allied Health Literature).

Some institutions have access to full-text journal databases, such as PsychARTICLES or ScienceDirect. These are produced by publishing companies (e.g., the American

Psychological Association and Elsevier, respectively) and only contain articles published in their own journals. Furthermore, as the Internet has become an integral part of everyday life for most of us, and researchers in particular, search engines such as Google have developed enormously. Google has created an academic search engine, Google Scholar, which can be useful in the very early stages of conducting a literature review or identifying a research question. It can provide a 'quick and dirty' way of exploring a potential area of study. It is also useful for locating full citations for articles if details of title or author have been lost. However, the utility of Google Scholar for anything more systematic is limited because Google has yet to publish its source of data or update frequency, which means it is impossible to know what is being searched and therefore what is potentially missing. Hence, the best way of ensuring a literature review is both thorough and systematic is to use a range of bibliographical databases.

Each bibliographical database has developed its own set of thesaurus terms or subject headings, which it uses for indexing individual journal articles. Consequently, employing the thesaurus terms used by the database being searched will increase the effectiveness of the search strategy. For example, MEDLINE has a series of Medical Subject Headings (MeSH headings); selecting the MeSH headings relevant to the question posed will optimize the likelihood of identifying relevant articles. For example, a review about South Asian men's experiences of an Early Intervention Service for psychosis may include the following MeSH terms in a MEDLINE search strategy: "Early Intervention (Education)", "Psychotic Disorders", "Perceptual Disorders" and "Hallucinations". These terms may seem inappropriate or may have been superseded by others in contemporary literature, but they will still be the most successful at identifying relevant articles in MEDLINE because this is how individual articles are indexed. Nevertheless, as suggested above, it may be appropriate to add terms introduced to the literature more recently or terms that better reflect the approach being taken in the current work. Whichever bibliographical database(s) is used, the effectiveness of the search strategy will be increased by using the thesaurus terms developed by that database.

Thesaurus terms are also used to index research articles by methodology, for example, "Randomized Controlled Trial", "Health Care Surveys", "Cross-Sectional Studies", "Case Reports" and "Qualitative Research" (from MEDLINE). These terms can be used to develop a methodology filter. However, when searching for qualitative evidence, subject headings are not so successful largely because they are very limited ("Qualitative Research" was added to the MEDLINE index in 2003 and has restricted effectiveness because of its lack of specificity). A comparison of qualitative research filters using subject headings and free-text terms (words that appear anywhere in the record, e.g., title, keywords or abstract) showed that none of the qualitative research filter strategies tested had a particularly high rate of precision (Shaw et al., 2004). Nevertheless, what this study showed is that three broad terms are as good as 40 plus more detailed terms when searching for qualitative research. Therefore it is advisable to use the broad-based qualitative methodology filter developed by Grant (2000) when attempting to identify qualitative research. This includes the following free-text terms: "findings",

Table 2.2   Example of MEDLINE search strategy

Early Intervention (Education)	MeSH Heading
Psychotic Disorders	MeSH Heading
Perceptual Disorders	MeSH Heading
Hallucinations	MeSH Heading
findings	Free-text term
interview$ OR Interview	Free-text terms
qualitative	Free-text term
OR/1-7	Boolean instruction

"interview$"[1] , "qualitative". Table 2.2 illustrates what a MEDLINE search strategy for our example research question might look like.

Even when planning a project that will use qualitative methods exclusively, it is necessary to review the existing quantitative evidence. Hence, when conducting a search, it will be necessary to run it twice – first without the methodology filter and secondly with it so as to narrow down the search results to increase the likelihood of identifying qualitative research.

When using a bibliographical database it is possible to save your search history, which is always advisable as it is likely that the process may be spread over several sessions. This will allow you to develop your strategy by testing out the effect of additional terms, by using different combinations of terms and, importantly, it also means you can return to your search and re-run it at a later date so as to update your records. In addition, most databases now enable you to download your search results either to a file or to a bibliographical software package, such as Endnote or Reference Manager. This will facilitate the screening phase of the review and facilitate later access to references when preparing manuscripts.

Screening search results and obtaining full-text articles

Screening records retrieved can be an onerous task. Another advantage of using bibliographical software is that it enables initial electronic screening; by ordering records by title it is possible to identify and discard duplicates quickly (it is advisable to make a working copy of the full original results so that anything discarded is not permanently deleted). For the sake of this illustration, let us assume we are conducting a review of

---

[1] The dollar sign, '$', in this example is a 'wildcard' used on MEDLINE. Most bibliographical databases use wildcards to broaden the utility of the search term; details of what different wildcards represent are usually available in the Help sections of databases. In this case, '$' is the symbol used in MEDLINE to denote the possibility of the additional letter, 's', so that it will retrieve records including both 'interview' and 'interviews'. In Web of Knowledge, the same function is denoted by '*' (e.g., "interview*" will retrieve "interview" and "interviews"; a dollar sign represents no character or one character and so will retrieve articles including the words, 'behaviour' and 'behavior' by using the term, "behavio$r"; and '?' denotes any single character so can identify 'woman' and 'women' by using the term, "wom?n".

qualitative evidence alone. Using bibliographical software it may be possible to identify and discard studies involving animals, for example, which are likely to be irrelevant to our example study about young South Asian men's experiences of Early Intervention Services for psychosis. You may then also search your records using terms that are likely to denote that a study is not relevant to your research question, such as "experiment", "child psychiatry", "women" and "female". The sensitivity of this electronic searching will depend on the software used; always err toward being over-inclusive when screening search results. Once those studies that are irrelevant are removed from the working database you can begin screening for eligibility, record by record, asking two questions: (i) is it relevant to my topic and (ii) does it use qualitative methods? The latter question is likely to be more challenging and it may be necessary to view the abstract or even the full-text article to determine whether the study employed qualitative methods.

Record keeping throughout your literature search is essential to ensure transparency, especially when conducting a search for the basis of a systematic review. A particularly useful way of recording the screening process is to use a PRISMA flowchart (Moher *et al.*, 2009).

Once the studies eligible for inclusion in your review have been identified, it is necessary to obtain them in full text. Most academic institutions and university hospitals have systems that link directly to bibliographical databases, meaning it is possible to click straight through to the appropriate journal (assuming the organization has a valid subscription), which will give you electronic access to the full-text article. If access to the article is not permitted, a copy can be obtained from the British Library using an Inter-Library Loan or document supply request.

Once all articles that are relevant to the research question have been identified it is necessary to conduct a quality appraisal. Further information on appraising the quality of qualitative research can be found in Chapter 16.

Synthesizing Qualitative Evidence

A number of methods for synthesizing qualitative evidence have been developed. This section focuses on one of those methods, meta-ethnography (Noblit & Hare, 1988). It then discusses some of the issues involved in conducting a meta-synthesis of qualitative evidence.

A very short history of the development of meta-synthesis

As we have seen, the function of systematic reviews of RCTs is to determine the effectiveness of interventions, whether those interventions involve a drug or a complex behavioural or educational programme. If data from the original studies are sufficiently homogeneous, then it is possible to conduct a meta-analysis so that levels of effectiveness between trials can be compared. This process involves amalgamating data from the original studies for further statistical analysis. This sort of integrative synthesis usually concerns theories of causality that make claims about generalizability, for example, about which types of intervention appear most likely to result in better identification of triggers for and management of symptoms of psychosis. The focus of an *integrative synthesis* has been described as: '*summarising data*, [..] where the concepts (or variables) under which data are to be summarised are assumed to be largely secure and well specified' (Dixon-Woods *et al.*, 2005, p. 46; emphasis in original). By contrast, an *interpretative synthesis* is involved with 'the development of concepts, and with the development and specification of theories that integrate those concepts' (Dixon-Woods *et al.*, 2005, p. 46). As such, in an interpretative synthesis it is unusual for concepts to be specified in advance; rather, they are developed through an interpretative analysis which is grounded in empirical data and conclusions from the original studies included in the synthesis. Rather than two distinct types of synthesis it is useful to look at integrative and interpretative synthesis techniques along a continuum, with some being largely (or wholly) integrative (e.g., a meta-analysis of interventions testing a new psychiatric drug for treating psychosis) and others being primarily interpretative (e.g., a meta-synthesis of qualitative studies investigating South Asian men's experience of an Early Intervention Service for psychosis).

The choice of synthesis method should first and foremost depend on the review question. If this involves making a judgement about and developing a theoretical understanding of the current knowledge base, then an interpretative synthesis will be necessary. By comparison, if the objective is to identify and describe current evidence, then an integrative synthesis will be most appropriate. What has become known as 'qualitative meta-synthesis' – and more recently, simply 'meta-synthesis' – a term coined by Stern and Harris (1985), sits toward the interpretative end of the spectrum alongside narrative summary, meta-ethnography (Noblit & Hare, 1988), meta-narrative mapping (Greenhalgh, 2004) and grounded theory (Strauss & Corbin, 1998) approaches to synthesis; at the integrative end of the continuum are content analysis, qualitative comparative analysis and Bayesian meta-analysis (for more details on each of these methods of synthesis see Dixon-Woods *et al.*, 2005; for a summary of key issues involved in methods of qualitative synthesis see Walsh & Downe, 2005).

Carrying out meta-synthesis

Meta-synthesis is 'research of research' (Paterson *et al.*, 2001, p. 5) which uses existing research publications as its primary data. This section includes an example of a qualitative meta-synthesis to illustrate the processes involved and to demonstrate the finished product. Probably the most influential method for synthesizing qualitative research is meta-ethnography; the example presented is a meta-ethnography of patients'[2] experience of managing antidepressants by Malpass *et al.* (2009).

Meta-ethnography   Meta-ethnography is a well-known interpretative method of synthesizing qualitative evidence developed by Noblit and Hare (1988). Indeed, it has become a model on which later syntheses have been based (e.g., Campbell *et al.*, 2003;

---

[2] This is the term used by the authors of the study.

Paterson *et al.*, 1998; Walter *et al.*, 2004). Meta-ethnography, as its name suggests, was developed to synthesize a number of independent ethnographies within a similar substantive field. For a meta-ethnography the original studies must be comparable in terms of topic *and* method. Certainly, some have argued that for meta-ethnography to be employed, the primary studies included must adopt the same method (Walsh & Downe, 2005) although it is unclear whether this relates to the epistemological framework as a whole (i.e., methodology), or simply the methods of data collection and/or analysis. This issue has been raised because qualitative research is a somewhat pluralistic term including diverse methods such as interpretative phenomenological analysis (see Chapter 8) and discourse analysis (see Chapter 11) which align themselves with very different epistemologies. It is easy to imagine why synthesizing data that are analysed in different ways, for example as an expression of an individual's reality of an experience or as a social construction of performative discourse, would be particularly challenging. Thus, intuitively, meta-ethnography is less problematic the more similar the primary studies are in terms of methodology, which is best represented by the method of analysis. That said, Campbell *et al.* (2003) and Walters *et al.* (2004) are examples of meta-ethnographies of studies employing different methods, thereby demonstrating possibilities for development within this synthesis technique.

In their seminal work, Noblit and Hare (1988) described seven stages of synthesis:

1. getting started;
2. deciding what is relevant;
3. reading the studies;
4. determining how the studies are related;
5. translating studies into one another;
6. synthesizing translations; and
7. expressing the synthesis (for an in-depth reflective discussion of the methodological challenges of implementing the phases of meta-ethnography see Atkins *et al.*, 2008).

Malpass *et al.* (2009; Table 2.3) follow the phases of synthesis outlined by Noblit and Hare (1988) but focus on identifying how papers are related, translating second order constructs into one another, synthesizing translations and expressing the synthesis. They also provide a useful summary of key terminology and procedures involved in meta-ethnography. First, Malpass *et al.* (2009) define first, second and third order constructs: *first order constructs* are interpretations of experience (e.g., service users' views, accounts and interpretations of their experiences of using antidepressants); *second order constructs* are interpretations of interpretations of experience (e.g., authors' views and interpretations of service users' views of antidepressants expressed as themes and concepts); *third order constructs* are interpretations of interpretations of interpretations of experience, representing a triple hermeneutic (e.g., views and interpretations of the synthesis team expressed in themes and key concepts). Secondly, they offer a clear explanation of the varying appropriateness of three translational synthesis techniques described by Noblit and Hare (1988): *reciprocal translational synthesis* is conducted when concepts of one study could be easily encompassed by those of another; *refutational*

Table 2.3   Summary of a meta-ethnography

Review question

What does the qualitative evidence tell us about patients' views of antidepressants for depression?

Method

Meta-ethnography

Search strategy

Databases: MEDLINE, Embase, CINAHL, Web of Science and PsycINFO

Phase 1: Scoping exercise using SPICE (Setting Perspective Intervention Comparison Evaluation tool; Booth, 2003) to refine search terms. Final search terms are included in the paper

Phase 2: Search of literature between 1990 and June 2007 (scoping exercise confirmed that earlier timeframes retrieved no further papers)

Phase 3: Reference lists of all potentially relevant papers were examined and reviewers wrote to authors of included papers asking them to identify additional relevant papers written by themselves or colleagues

Screening

AM screened all titles and abstracts and AS and DK screened a subset using the questions: 'Is this qualitative research?' and 'Is this paper relevant to the meta-ethnography?' Papers were excluded if they did not use qualitative methods and if they were irrelevant to the review question (e.g., if they focused on experiences of depression and not antidepressants, on GPs' experiences of antidepressants, or the use of antidepressants for a mental illness other than depression)

Method of appraisal

Three methods of appraisal were piloted: (1) a modified version of CASP (Critical Appraisal Skills Programme checklist for qualitative research; Public Health Resource Unit, 1998); (2) a Quality Framework produced by the National Centre for Social Research (2003); (3) and an iterative guide to quality developed by Mays and Pope (2000)

A modified version of CASP was used; this excluded the use of a scoring system and adopted the framework developed by Dixon-Woods *et al.* (2007) to determine whether a paper was a key paper (KP), satisfactory (SAT), of questionable quality (?), irrelevant (IRR) or methodologically fatally flawed (FF)

Appraisal was not used to exclude papers but to test the contributions they made. Reviewers were interested to determine whether the synthesis would remain the same if only key papers were included

Phases of synthesis

Phase 1: Read and re-read original papers in chronological order noting the second order constructs (or themes) reported

Phase 2: Tables of second order constructs were compiled (by AM and AS) including raw data from original papers (i.e., first order constructs) and any comments about the papers. Conceptual maps were also drawn for each paper to illustrate how the major second order constructs were related to each other in order to preserve the contextual meanings of the original study

---

Table 2.3   *(Continued)*

Review question

Phase 3: Translating studies into one another. AM created a spreadsheet to include all second order constructs for each paper in turn. Original authors' own language (or close paraphrase) was used. This spreadsheet was then used to conduct a comparison of conceptual terms used across studies. This involves an interpretative reading of meaning but not further conceptual development. A table was created to record the outcome of this translation process

Phase 4: Synthesizing translations. Papers were split into two groups: (1) papers about the decision-making process; and (2) papers representing four 'moral' junctures related to antidepressants. A reciprocal synthesis of these two groups was conducted. These were then drawn together in a line of argument synthesis

Results

Tables including the characteristics of original papers and the results of the translation process were included. Diagrams of the reciprocal synthesis and line of argument synthesis were included

Findings were presented as a series of themes with extracts of raw data (first order constructs) cited in original papers and the original authors' commentary

Notes

A challenge relating to the theoretical or methodological perspectives of original papers was highlighted. Reviewers noted that those who adopt a relativist stance argue that synthesizing qualitative studies with different epistemologies is not desirable or feasible because each study represents a different view influenced by differences in theory or method. Nevertheless, reviewers rejected this limitation because original studies included in this synthesis that declared their epistemological framework adopted a symbolic interactionist perspective and so were in line theoretically. Reviewers note the benefits of multiple reviewers independently reading original papers and identifying second order constructs because it is these constructs that form the bedrock of the synthesis

There was no effect on the synthesis when all papers except those rated as key papers were excluded. Reviewers concluded that testing the contribution of papers was an effective use of the critical appraisal process

Source: Malpass, A., Shaw, A., Sharp, D., *et al.* (2009). "Medication career" or "Moral career"? The two sides of managing antidepressants: A meta-ethnography of patients' experience of antidepressants. *Social Science & Medicine, 68*, 154–168.

translational synthesis is where concepts are contested across papers; and *lines of argument synthesis* is used when different studies investigate different aspects of the same phenomenon and the synthesis is conducted to create a fuller picture of the phenomenon by employing metaphors from original studies to construct an argument about what the set of papers as a whole can tell us. These techniques may be conducted in series or just those that are 'fit for purpose' will be employed. For example, Malpass *et al.* (2009) do not carry out a refutational translational synthesis because the original studies included in their review had fairly homogeneous findings making that process unnecessary (see the full-text article of Malpass *et al.*'s meta-ethnography for details).

Issues to consider when synthesizing qualitative evidence

There are some key issues that need to be considered when synthesizing qualitative literature. First, reviewers must make a decision about how primary studies will be appraised; secondly, a decision about whether the quality appraisal will determine the inclusion or exclusion of original studies or whether a critical evaluation of papers will run throughout the whole process, as Dixon-Woods *et al.* (2006) advise, is required. The outcome of this second decision has implications for how qualitative meta-synthesis fits within the existing hierarchy of evidence framework. Of course we want qualitative evidence to contribute to evidence-based practice but, for that to happen, our synthesis techniques need to be reflexive and critical to ensure the trustworthiness of findings applied in practice (see Chapter 16).

There is also a clear need for the interpretative activity involved in a qualitative meta-synthesis to be transparent. Lincoln and Guba (1985) highlight the significance of the hermeneutic and dialectic processes within meta-synthesis; just as primary qualitative analysts must be aware of their presuppositions, reviewers who synthesize qualitative evidence need to engage in reflexive work. Furthermore, because meta-synthesis is usually carried out by a team of reviewers, that team needs to be transparent about its procedures and interactions: the review team needs to elaborate the procedures implemented to identify and appraise original papers; it needs to discuss the original papers in depth; and at every stage of the synthesis it needs to think through its interpretations and document its discussions to ensure the findings and conclusions of the original studies are represented in a fair and appropriate manner. As much as the interpretative qualitative analysis of interview data involves a double hermeneutic (Smith *et al.*, 2009), a synthesis of qualitative evidence involves a triple hermeneutic: as described above, a synthesis of qualitative evidence involves interpretations of interpretations of interpretations (Malpass *et al.*, 2009).

Finally, as Bondas and Hall (2007) have suggested, meta-synthesis may not be for the faint hearted. There are many epistemological, ontological and methodological issues which intertwine to make qualitative meta-synthesis a challenging pursuit. As outlined above, questions around the appropriateness of synthesizing original studies that employ different methods or that are based upon distinct epistemologies remain. One could argue that synthesizing studies that have used a social constructionist discourse analysis and those that have adopted a symbolic interactionist framework, using a method such as interpretative phenomenological analysis, pose similar problems as those faced when attempting to synthesize quantitative and qualitative evidence. Mixing different qualitative methods can create as many epistemological challenges as mixing quantitative and qualitative methods. A Pragmatic approach, as proposed by Yardley and Bishop (2008), offers a way of dealing with what may appear to be insurmountable epistemological differences. Instead of framing the definition of knowledge within natural science which evokes a positivist stance toward objectivity and a preference for the scientific method (i.e., experiments), Pragmatism proposes that science and common sense alike can contribute to valid knowledge. Thus, qualitative research, which often aligns itself with human science (for a detailed discussion of what constitutes human science see Polkinghorne, 1998) can, within a Pragmatic approach, contribute to what is considered valid scientific knowledge.

As the body of evidence from which we are working becomes increasingly heterogeneous, it is imperative that we develop systematic reviewing methodology that can not only deal with that diversity but that also synthesizes the evidence base on the grounds that 'valid scientific knowledge' can take many forms. Indeed, the significance of qualitative meta-synthesis to evidence-based practice is summarized by Flemming: 'Developers of policy and practice need to be able to understand the kind of tensions that exist between the effectiveness of interventions and their implementation in practice and need to be able to reference an evidence base that has systematically drawn on diverse sources of evidence to enable them do this' (Flemming, 2010, p. 151).

To conclude, this chapter has summarized the procedures involved in identifying and synthesizing qualitative research literature. It is to be hoped it has provided some useful tips and some food for thought for developing future research ventures.

References

Atkins, S., Lewin, S., Smith, H., Engel, M., Fretheim, A. & Volmink, J. (2008). Conducting a meta-ethnography of qualitative literature: Lessons learnt. *BMC Medical Research Methodology*, *8*, 21. Retrieved 16 February 2010 from http://www.biomedcentral.com/1471-2288/8/21.

Bondas, T. & Hall, E.O.C. (2007). Challenges in approaching metasynthesis research. *Qualitative Health Research*, *17*, 113–121.

Booth, A. (2003). Formulating answerable questions. In A. Booth & A. Brice (Eds.)*Evidence based practice: A handbook for information professionals* (pp. 59–66). London: Facet.

Buckland, M.K. & Gey, F. (1994). The relationship between recall and precision. *Journal of the American Society for Information Retrieval*, *45*, 12–19.

Campbell, R., Pound, P., Pope, C., Britten, N., Pill, R., Morgan, M., *et al.* (2003). Evaluating meta-ethnography: A synthesis of qualitative research on lay experiences of diabetes and diabetes care. *Social Science and Medicine*, *56*, 671–684.

Cochrane Collaboration. Retrieved 29 January 2010 from http://www.cochrane.org/.

Cochrane Qualitative Research Methods Group. (CQRMG). Retrieved 14 June 2010 from http://www.joannabriggs.edu.au/cqrmg/about.html.

Department of Health. (2008). Increasing Access to Psychological Therapies Programme (IAPT) Commissioning Toolkit. London: Department of Health. Retrieved 14 June 2010 from http://www.dh.gov.uk/en/Publicationsandstatistics/Publications/PublicationsPolicyAnd Guidance/DH_084065.

Diagnostic Strategies for Information Retrieval. (2004). Quantitative issues in information retrieval. Retrieved 29 January 2010 from http://www.diagnosticstrategies.com/info_retrieval.htm.

Dixon-Woods, M., Agarwal, S., Jones, D., Young, B. & Sutton, A. (2005). Synthesising qualitative and quantitative evidence. *Journal of Health Services Research and Policy*, *10*, 45–53.

Dixon-Woods, M., Cavers, D., Agarwal, S., Annandale, E., Arthur, A., Harvey, J., *et al.* (2006). Conducting a critical interpretive synthesis of the literature on access to healthcare by vulnerable groups. *BMC Medical Research Methodology*, *6*, 35. Retrieved 1 February 2010 from http://www.biomedcentral.com/1471-2288/6/35.

Dixon-Woods, M., Fitzpatrick, R. & Roberts, K. (2001). Including qualitative research in systematic reviews: opportunities and problems. *Journal of Evaluation in Clinical Practice, 7,* 125–133.

Dixon-Woods, M., Sutton, A., Shaw, R., Miller, T., Smith, J., Young, B., *et al.* (2007). Appraising qualitative research for inclusion in systematic reviews: a quantitative and qualitative comparison of three methods. *Journal of Health Services Research and Policy, 12,* 42–47.

Elliott, R., Fischer, C.T. & Rennie, D.L. (1999). Evolving guidelines for publication of qualitative research studies in psychology and related fields. *British Journal of Clinical Psychology, 38,* 215–229.

Flemming, K. (2010). The use of morphine to treat cancer-related pain: A synthesis of quantitative and qualitative research. *Journal of Pain and Symptom Management, 39,* 139–154.

Golsworthy, R. & Coyle, A. (2001). Practitioners accounts of religious and spiritual dimensions in bereavement therapy. *Counselling Psychology Quarterly, 14,* 183–202.

Grant, M.J. (2000). *Searching for qualitative research studies on the MEDLINE database: The development of an optimal search strategy.* Aberystwyth, University of Wales: Department of Information and Library Studies.

Greenhalgh, T. (2004). Meta-narrative mapping: A new approach to the synthesis of complex evidence. In B. Hurwitz, T. Greenhalgh & V. Skultans (Eds.) *Narrative research in health and illness* 349–381). London: BMJ Publications.

Guyatt, G.H., Meade, M.O., Jaeschke, R.Z., Cook, D.J. & Haynes, R.B. (2000). Practitioners of evidence based care. *British Medical Journal, 320,* 954–955.

Kroenke K. & Spitzer, R.L. (2002). The PHQ-9: A new depression diagnostic and severity measure. *Psychiatric Annals, 32,* 509–521.

Larkin, M., Clifton, E. & De Visser, R. (2009). Making sense of 'consent' in a constrained environment. *International Journal of Law and Psychiatry, 32,* 176–183.

Lincoln, Y.S. & Guba, E.G. (1985). Establishing trustworthiness. In Y.S. Lincoln & E.G. Guba (Eds.) *Naturalistic inquiry* 289–331). Newbury Park, CA: Sage.

Malpass, A., Shaw, A., Sharp, D., Walter, F., Feder, G., Ridd, M., *et al.* (2009). "Medication career" or "Moral career"? The two sides of managing antidepressants: A meta-ethnography of patients' experience of antidepressants. *Social Science and Medicine, 68,* 154–168.

Marks, D.F. & Sykes, C.M. (2004). Synthesising evidence: systematic reviews, meta-analysis and preference analysis. In D.F. Marks & L. Yardley (Eds.) *Research methods for clinical and health psychology* 185–209). London: Sage.

Martindale, S.J., Chambers, E. & Thompson, A.R. (2009). Clinical psychology service users' experiences of confidentiality and informed consent: A qualitative analysis. *Psychology and Psychotherapy: Theory, Research and Practice, 82,* 355–368.

Mays, N. & Pope, C. (2000). Qualitative research in health care: Assessing quality in qualitative research. *British Medical Journal, 320,* 50–52.

Midgley, N., Target, M. & Smith, J.A. (2006). The outcome of child psychoanalysis from the patient's point of view: A qualitative analysis of a long-term follow-up study. *Psychology and Psychotherapy: Theory, Research and Practice, 79,* 257–269.

Moher, D., Liberati, A., Tetzlaff, J., Altman, D.G.; PRISMA Group (2009). Preferred reporting items for systematic reviews and meta-analyses: The PRISMA Statement. *PLoS Med, 6,* e1000097. doi: 10.1371/journal.pmed1000097. Retrieved 29 January 2010 from http://www.prisma-statement.org.

Mulrow, C., Langhorne, P. & Grimshaw, J. (1997). Integrating heterogeneous pieces of evidence in systematic reviews. *Annals of Internal Medicine, 127,* 989–995.

National Centre for Social Research. (2003). *Quality in qualitative evaluation: A framework for assessing research evidence.* London: National Centre for Social Research/Cabinet Office.

NHS Centre for Reviews and Dissemination. (2001). *Undertaking systematic reviews of research on effectiveness: CRD's guidance for those carrying out or commissioning reviews.* Report Number 4 (2nd edn). York: CRD.

NICE (2008). Cognitive behavioural therapy for the management of common mental health problems. Commissioning Guide: implementing NICE guidance. London: NICE. Retrieved 14 June 2010 from http://www.nice.org.uk/usingguidance/commissioningguides/cognitive behaviouraltherapyservice/cbt.jsp.

Noblit, G. & Hare, R. (1988). *Meta-ethnography: Synthesising qualitative studies.* Newbury Park, CA: Sage.

O'Rourke, A., Booth, A. & Ford, N. (1999). Another fine MeSH: clinical medicine meets information science. *Journal of Information Science, 25,* 275–281.

Paterson, B., Thorne, S. & Dewis, M. (1998). Adapting to and managing diabetes. *Journal of Nursing Scholarship, 30,* 57–62.

Paterson, B.L., Thorne, S.E., Canam, C. & Jillings, C. (2001). *Meta-study of qualitative health research: A practical guide to meta-analysis and meta-synthesis.* Thousand Oaks, CA: Sage.

Polkinghorne, D.E. (1988). *Narrative knowing and the human sciences.* Albany, NY: SUNY.

Public Health Resource Unit (PHRU). (1998). Critical appraisal skills programme (CASP). Retrieved 9 February 2010 from http://www.phru.nhs.uk/Pages/PHD/resources.htm.

Shaw, R.L. (2010). Conducting literature reviews. In M. Forrester (Ed.) *Doing qualitative research in psychology: A practical guide* (pp.39–52). London: Sage.

Shaw, R.L., Booth, A., Sutton, A.J., Miller, T., Smith, J.A., Young, B., *et al.* (2004). Finding qualitative research: An evaluation of search strategies. *BMC Medical Research Methodology, 4* (5). Retrieved 29 January 2010 from http://www.biomedcentral.com/1471-2288/4/5.

Smith, J.A., Flowers, P. & Larkin, M. (2009). *Interpretative phenomenological analysis: Theory, method and research.* London: Sage.

Stern, P.N. & Harris C.C. (1985). Women's health and the self-care paradox: A model to guide self-care readiness. *Health Care for Women International, 6,* 151–163.

Strauss, A. & Corbin, J. (1998). *The basics of qualitative research: Techniques and procedures for developing Grounded Theory* (2nd edn). Thousand Oaks, CA: Sage.

Walsh, D. & Downe, S. (2005). Meta-synthesis method for qualitative research: A literature review. *Journal of Advanced Nursing, 50,* 204–211.

Walter, F.M., Emery, J., Braithwaite, D. & Marteau, T.M. (2004). Lay understanding of familial risk of common chronic diseases: A systematic review and synthesis of qualitative research. *Annals of Family Medicine, 2,* 583–594.

Yardley, L. & Bishop, F. (2008). Mixing qualitative and quantitative methods: A Pragmatic approach. In W. Stainton Rogers & C. Willig (Eds.) *The SAGE handbook of qualitative research in psychology* 352–370). London: Sage.

Further reading and useful website

Dixon-Woods, M., Bonas, S., Booth, A., Jones, D.R., Miller, T.A., Shaw, R.L., *et al.* (2006) How can systematic qualitative reviews incorporate qualitative research? A critical perspective. *Qualitative Research, 6,* 27–44.

School of Health and Related Research (ScHARR), University of Sheffield: http://www.shef.ac.uk/scharr/index.html.

Walsh, D. & Downe, S. (2005). Meta-synthesis method for qualitative research: A literature review. *Journal of Advanced Nursing, 50,* 204–211.

3

Ethical Issues in Qualitative Mental Health Research

Andrew R. Thompson and Eleni Chambers

Introduction: Codes, Principles and Laws are Useful but it is About Judgement and Everyday Practice

This chapter seeks to raise awareness of the specific ethical dilemmas that mental health practitioners may encounter when conducting qualitative research, and to discuss how best to address these issues in the context of greater involvement with service users and members of the public. Qualitative research within this arena can raise a number of specific issues and dilemmas (not least how to balance holding multiple roles such as practitioner and researcher or service user and researcher), and this chapter addresses the following areas:

- ethical principles in relation to the general conduct of research;
- the specific ethical issues and dilemmas that need to be considered when conducting qualitative research in mental health; and
- discussion of how such issues might be addressed.

The majority of mental health qualitative research has involved the use of interviews and we focus mainly upon the ethical issues associated with this form of data collection in this chapter, although many of the issues we discuss will also be pertinent to qualitative research more generally.

There is a relative dearth of empirical studies in this area that actually identify what the issues might be for participants and researchers. However, numerous discussion articles outline the need for specific consideration of issues in relation to: informed consent and self-determination; confidentiality and privacy; avoiding harm; dual-role

Qualitative Research Methods in Mental Health and Psychotherapy: A Guide for Students and Practitioners, First Edition. Edited by D. Harper and A.R. Thompson.
© 2012 John Wiley & Sons, Ltd. Published 2012 by John Wiley & Sons, Ltd.

and over-involvement; and politics and power (for reviews of this area see Allmark *et al.*, 2009; Graham *et al.*, 2006; Thompson & Russo, in press). We cover all of these issues below in some detail, but prior to doing this we will first introduce the broader concept of ethics.

'Ethics' refers to moral principles that guide action and are essentially derived from philosophical theories. The two positions most often discussed being the *deontological and consequentialist* positions. Put very simply, deontological theories place emphasis on the importance of carrying out good actions, in accordance with moral rules or duties, with rights-based theories being an example of this. Consequentialist theories emphasize the importance of achieving good consequences when deciding what to do, utilitarianism being the most widely known type of consequentialism (see Francis, 2009).

In an attempt to resolve some of the difficulties that arise from translating the above philosophical positions into actual practice that is accepted by a wide number of people the *principles* approach has arisen. This is essentially a set of fundamental moral rules and it is worth stating that most professional codes largely build upon the four ethical principles of:

- *Respect for autonomy*: respecting an individual's right to make decisions and enabling them to make reasoned informed choices.
- *Beneficence*: seeking to achieve the best balance between risk and benefit that achieves the greatest benefits for the individual.
- *Non-maleficence*: avoiding causing harm.
- *Justice*: addressing issues fairly for individuals in the same or similar situation (Beauchamp & Childress, 2001).

The limitations of the principles approach laid out above are well established and centre upon the principles being: first, fairly obvious and therefore failing to add anything to common clinical/research sense; and, secondly, that they often conflict with one another and as such rarely offer a solution to more complex ethical dilemmas. For example, conflicts can arise between the principles of autonomy and beneficence when deciding whether it is necessary to breach confidentiality where the risk of potential self-harm has been disclosed during data collection.

Consequently, as is widely acknowledged by authors of most codes, engaging with ethical issues is not a simple matter of adhering to professional guidelines and regulations, or even identifying and engaging with specific ethical dilemmas (each of which will have its own unique social, theoretical and political context). Alternatively, we hope to show that it is more useful to view ethics as part of everyday research (and professional) practice, with the focus being on relationships and emotions, and on reasoned judgement – informed by guidelines and laws.

Clearly, professional codes of practice of mental health practitioners contain some guidance, although they are highly variable in the extent that they specifically cover research practice. It should go without saying that researchers understand and adhere to their professional codes and the codes of national health and social care providers (e.g., American Psychological Association, 2010; British Association of Social Workers, 2002; British Psychological Society, 2005, 2006; Department of Health, 2005; Health Professions Council, 2008; Nursing and Midwifery Council, 2010).

We will not endeavour to describe in any detail the codes of any one particular professional group here as they all essentially have some limitations, and it is worth searching more widely than your own professional base when negotiating a particular issue as this can facilitate further reflection. For example, some professional bodies have produced additional guidance on specific topics such as conducting research: with people in the NHS; where capacity to consent may be an issue; and conducting research on the Internet (e.g., British Psychological Society, 2005, 2007, 2008).

Prior to outlining some of the specific ethical issues that might be encountered in undertaking qualitative research, it will be useful to undertake a brief review of the history of ethical research review as this sets the context for some of the nuanced issues we go on to discuss.

Ethical Review: Moving Towards Inclusive Practice

The first significant attempt to develop a formal code of practice to guide research followed the trials at the end of the Second World War of the Nazi doctors who had conducted gross experimentation on people against their will. This led to the 10-point Nuremberg Code and later to the World Medical Association Declaration of Helsinki in 1964 (World Medical Association, 2002).

Understandably, given the background to the development of these codes, the principle of preventing harm to research participants taking part in medical studies arguably became the central concern for those reviewing applications to conduct health and social care research. Of course this remains of the uppermost importance and is still at the heart of most guidance and codes. For example, the Research Governance Framework for Health and Social Care in the UK is explicit in stating 'The dignity, rights, safety and well-being of participants must be the primary consideration in any research study' (Department of Health, 2005, p. 7). The American Psychological Association has also recently amended its ethical code, following issues of military psychologists being involved in inhumane interrogation practices, to make it clear that that maintenance of human rights is the fundamental principle that should be upheld (American Psychological Association, 2010).

In the United Kingdom, there has for a number of years been a division between ethical review and research governance, at least in health care. This commenced with the Department of Health, largely in response to a number of biomedical ethical scandals (e.g., Bristol Royal Infirmary Inquiry, 2001; Royal Liverpool Children's Inquiry, 2001) putting together the Research Governance Framework for Health and Social Care in 2001 (Department of Health, 2005). This framework systematically covers all aspects of research including checking whether ethical scrutiny has occurred, financial probity, health and safety, and the responsibilities of all stakeholders.

The National Research Ethics Service (NRES), launched in 2007, built on the system of Local Research Ethics Committees established in 1991 (Department of Health, 1991) to provide a standardized framework and process for obtaining ethical scrutiny across health and, more recently, social care research. The processes and procedures associated with ethical review have continued to evolve over recent years largely to address a number of concerns.

Several commentators have discussed the constraining and paternalistic nature of traditional biomedical ethical procedures and suggested that such procedures are a form of 'ethics creep' into psychosocial research (Haggerty, 2004, p. 391; Holland, 2007). Indeed, it has been suggested that the application of simple and inflexible ethical codes has led to an objectification of ethics, where ethical issues might simply be viewed as a set of procedural tasks to be dealt with before research commences, and this is extremely dangerous as it might serve to switch off the novice researcher from engaging with ethics in an ongoing reflexive fashion (Small, 2001).

In response to a recent Department of Health consultation on ethical review, INVOLVE, the advisory group set up to promote and support public involvement in health and social care (see www.invo.org.uk), responded: 'We are aware of a number of research proposals which we regarded as having good quality involvement that have encountered difficulties because of the perceptions of Research Ethics Committees (RECs) as to the vulnerability and capability of the active participants. What those committees have probably regarded as appropriate protective considerations have often been seen by those who are the subject of ethic review decisions as being overly paternalistic, ill informed, and disempowering' (INVOLVE, 2004, p. 1).

There have been relatively few studies exploring the ethical priorities of service users in relation to mental health research. Carrick (2006) conducted a Delphi study to look at the views of service users and one of her main findings was that service users were very keen for higher levels of involvement in ethical review.

Recently, the NRES and INVOLVE have produced a joint statement to provide clarity and guidance on patient and public involvement in research and the requirements of research ethics review. This statement makes it very clear that research should involve members of the research population early on in the consideration of ethical issues. It goes on to clarify, in an attempt to encourage early involvement, that ethical approval is not needed for involvement in research planning, even if people are recruited from the NHS (NRES and INVOLVE, 2009).

In addition, there is now a focus upon NHS ethics and governance committees to have qualitative research expertise and to have a range of lay members drawn from a wide variety of backgrounds (see Department of Health, 2007). Consequently, a wider range of professionals, service users and members of the public have come onto ethics committees over recent years and are beginning to address some of the concerns raised by earlier commentators.

However, problems still remain with parts of the system, particularly with relation to governance procedures. Individual Health Care Trusts have largely developed their own procedures, many of which seem inappropriate for qualitative research and unnecessarily unwieldy for social science research more generally. This has led some to call for a streamlining of the processes associated with implementation of the governance framework, and others to call for it to be abolished altogether (Goodacre, 2010).

Awareness of the historical backdrop to the development of ethical codes is important in understanding some of the reasons for what has until relatively recently been seen by many as a paternalistic and perhaps *overly protective* system of ethical review, which has largely located the ability to make decisions solely with professionals. Fortunately, the move towards greater service user and public involvement in ethics procedures has begun to redress this balance and we are now in a position where it is widely acknowledged that: '[i]t is good practice and the Research Ethics Committee (REC) will look more favourably upon your application if you involve patients and representatives of the group likely to be recruited' (NRES, 2009, p. 6).

The message is clear: early involvement of the potential research population in the development of research protocols or proposals is important in facilitating both good ethical research practice and smooth movement through the various ethical procedures that exist.

It is also essential that any proposed research plans are sufficiently rigorous and the chapters elsewhere in this book outline some of the key ingredients necessary in ensuring that this aim is achieved. It is always good practice (if not a requirement) that peers and supervisors review protocols prior to formal submission to ethical and governance committees. Where opportunities exist to attend an ethics committee review meeting, these should always be accepted, as they provide an opportunity to learn and discuss issues in greater depth than will usually be provided in feedback letters. Electronic resources such as the Research Ethics Guidebook and the National Research Ethics Service also provide essential information for guiding seasoned and novice researchers alike through the necessary (and often complex) processes (see further reading box that concludes this chapter).

Vulnerable Participants and Sensitive Topics: Recognizing That We Are All Vulnerable

Many ethical guidelines, commentators and other authors on the ethical process have often described participants from mental health settings (amongst others) as 'vulnerable' and the topics likely to be explored as 'sensitive' (e.g., Liamputtong, 2007).

Such terms as vulnerable and sensitive are easily taken for granted and it is worth unpacking them a little before we progress. The use of such terms risks participants of mental health research (in particular, service users) becoming disempowered through placing emphasis on a perceived need for protection which relates back to the paternalistic researcher stance already described. However, as Davison (2004) has stated in relation to qualitative research conducted in the social work arena: 'The capacity for harm is incumbent in any research – vulnerability and conflicting emotions can be linking experiences for both the research informant and the researcher' (p. 381).

The important point here is that both researcher and researched are vulnerable, indeed, we are all soft tissued organisms with emotions, and as such are vulnerable in certain situations or contexts to both physical and psychological harm. It is for the researcher to reflect on in what way the specific context of their proposed study might create vulnerability, rather than for the research team to assume that a particular group is vulnerable per se on the basis of their membership of a particular group or because they have particular characteristics (Jenkins, 2008). Rosenblatt (1995) has discussed some of these issues in relation to carrying out bereavement research; distress is to be expected in discussing such topics with participants and the researcher needs to be practiced in staying with emotional subjects and facilitating participant choice as to whether to continue.

Further, exploration of the construction of particular groups status as 'marginalized', 'stigmatized' or 'vulnerable' is in itself a worthy focus of qualitative research as we shall see in the later chapters. Therefore, having a starting position of seeing a group as inherently vulnerable or sensitive is clearly theoretically at odds with such constructionist and critical approaches (see, for example, the Critical Psychiatry Website).

Further arguments against the labelling of groups of participants should be only too familiar to many mental health practitioners in relation to the core principles they already use to guide their professional work (think anti-oppressive practice or normalization, e.g., Wolfensberger, 1972). The awareness of such theories should enable mental health researchers to understand the need to strive to create equal access to the procedures and practices without creating further devaluation by labelling specific groups as vulnerable per se. There may be a need to adapt procedures around, for example, gaining consent but this should always be done with such principles as normalization in mind. Again, this is an area where mental health practitioners may have pre-existing competencies in relation to assessing and understanding capacity to consent (British Psychological Society, 2008).

Researchers need to be equally aware of their own vulnerabilities whilst engaged in a study and they must finds ways of managing and understanding this. Davison (2004) discusses how supervision can have a particularly important role in assisting researchers to be open in exploring their emotional reactions and exploring the role this may have on the conduct of a study. This may call for a different type of supervision than is usually found in relation to quantitative research but may not be unfamiliar to mental health practitioners because of similarities with clinical supervision and reflexive practice. Recently, Gleeson has described a 'process model' for research supervision and contrasted this with the traditional 'progress model'. She advocates placing emphasis on facilitating reflection and learning rather than purely focusing on how to complete a particular task (Gleeson & Mortimore, 2010). In line with Davison's discussion, this model sees supervision as a place for exploring how pre-existing ideas, research conduct and so on, shapes a study.

Informed Consent and Respect for Autonomy

As already stated, the principle of respecting autonomy is central to ethical codes and connected to facilitating informed consent. Informed consent is achieved when the nature, purpose and consequence of the research are understood by would-be participants. Consequently, it covers not only consent forms and information sheets, but adequate awareness of research aims, methods, sources of funding, conflicts of interest, affiliations of the researchers and potential risks–benefits (World Medical Association, 2002).

There is now much helpful practical advice on achieving informed consent and explicit recommendations to involve members of the research population in developing the recruitment procedures (see Further reading box).

We have already mentioned capacity issues, and the Mental Capacity Act (2005) in the United Kingdom has established a legal framework for people lacking the capacity to make decisions for themselves and this may need to be considered in planning strategies to facilitate opportunities for participants to provide informed consent. It may in some circumstances be necessary to carry out formal assessment of capacity; however, this is an area that needs careful consideration as there is evidence that formal assessments may reduce participation (Adamis et al., 2005). Further, there is a wider issue of being careful not to present barriers to participation.

Consent should not be seen as something that is necessarily simply gained once, and researchers need to use interpersonal skills to provide participants with opportunities to reaffirm (or not) their wish to continue in a study. So-called 'processual' or ongoing consent may be particularly important in conducting in-depth interviews with people, which may lead to participants finding themselves revealing information they had not considered in advance (we revisit this when we discuss privacy below).

Confidentiality and Privacy

There is an important distinction between privacy and confidentiality, with privacy relating to areas of life one wishes to keep private and confidentiality relating to the protection of private information that one has chosen to share for a specified reason (Allmark et al., 2009). A number of authors have commented on the potential for infringement into the privacy of non-consented individuals, as may be the case when asking about relationships, social support or treatment, and participants go on to talk about people other than themselves (e.g., Forbat & Henderson, 2003).

This raises all sorts of subtle ethical issues, such as how to manage the influence of relationship disclosures. Forbat and Henderson (2003) have discussed some of the nuances of this in relation to their research with people with a diagnosis of bipolar disorder and people identifying themselves as their carers. Clarification of the boundaries of the researcher–participant relationship is important as mental health practitioners will have requirements under their professional registration codes to report certain risks (such as child abuse), yet, as Forbat and Henderson discuss, the issues are often likely to be more subtle than disclosures of such risk, where the course of action is fairly well proscribed. Seeking advice from the potential research population as to how such issues might be resolved prior to commencing a study will greatly enhance a research team's ability to address such subtle issues as they arise.

A difficulty for qualitative studies is that the nature of the data that are obtained may allow others to reconstruct their identity despite safeguards such as the use of pseudonyms. There is a particular risk when participants are recruited from services or professional groups or small participant populations (i.e., in the sorts of settings and contexts that mental health practitioners and service user researchers primarily conduct qualitative research; Thompson & Russo, in press).

Consent should be sought to use material, and routine feedback to participants particularly of the excerpts that are to be reported should typically occur unless participants have expressly stated they do not wish this to happen. This is possible even with qualitative methods where there is an element of interpretation. For example, in a study conducted by Donnison et al. (2009) which explored communication within mental health teams, participants were sent all of the individual quotes that were to be used and asked to provide further consent for the use of the material.

Avoiding Harm

There is always the potential for any interaction to lead to harm, and participants in mental health qualitative studies face a number of potential risks (as do researchers). The risk most usually discussed is that of becoming upset whilst reflecting, sharing and recalling particular experiences.

There are relatively few empirical studies that have looked at the experience of participants of discussing emotionally charged topics. The literature that exists is equivocal – some studies indicate that participants can find the experience unsatisfactory but others report that participants found the experience to be beneficial in its own right (Ruzek & Zatzick, 2000; Scott et al., 2002). Graham et al. (2007) conducted 50 interviews with participants who had recently participated in NatCen (social policy) research and found that participants showed no aversion to discussing painful issues provided they felt the study was worthwhile.

Therefore, it is important to be mindful that experiencing distress is not necessarily experienced as harmful. Indeed, there is now substantial evidence that emotional disclosure across a range of settings has the potential to be beneficial. The point is that we need to be mindful of the potential for distress and practiced at managing it – but not necessarily to avoid it. The skilled researcher will be able to create an environment where a participant may become distressed and where they will feel enabled to choose whether or not to proceed with the interview.

Clearly, researchers should ensure that participants have space at the end of the interview to ensure that any emotional distress experienced during the interview has reduced, and that participants are aware of where they can access additional emotional support if required. Generally, it is good practice to offer sufficient post-interview space for reflection on the process to occur (Fossey et al., 2002).

Multiple Roles and Dual Relationships

Ethical issues may arise where researchers hold dual or even multiple roles – perhaps as a practitioner researcher, service user researcher, manager researcher or any combination of these roles. There may be subtle risks of coercion or conflicts of interests, such as where one party wishes to show a service in a particular light or has an 'axe to grind' about a particular type of intervention. Such conflicts will influence all aspects of a research study from the questions asked to the interpretations of the data obtained. Conversely, the competencies related to non-researcher roles may also confer transferable benefits to the research situation. The important point for researchers holding multiple roles is to be open to exploring in what ways these roles might lead to ethical dilemmas.

Brinkman and Kvale (2008) have commented that the ability to create a therapeutic alliance by practitioner researchers might also create implicit pressure on participants' ability to maintain boundaries of privacy. However, whilst this may pose a threat, 'participants may be far more discerning about the nature of research than researchers often give them credit for; to argue otherwise removes participant agency and control over what is revealed and withheld' (Clarke, 2006, p. 21).

A common criticism that service user researchers have faced is that they are potentially biased or run the risk of becoming over-involved (Sweeney et al., 2009). However, several studies have reported advantages, for example, Clarke et al. (1999) found that when mental health service users were dissatisfied with the services they had received they were more likely to disclose this to service user interviewers.

Conversely, some studies have reported disadvantages associated with the role of service user researcher. Bryant and Beckett (2006) found that user researchers tended not to explore issues as fully when carrying out interviews. They concluded this was because of the user researchers' relative inexperience in interviewing, a lack of probing perhaps because of an assumption that because they had a shared experience they understood the participants without having to explore issues more deeply and lack of exploration because they had not wanted to appear intrusive. The key issue here is not about service user researchers, but about all researchers developing sufficient competencies prior to engaging with participants (for further discussion of these issues in specific relation to service user research see Chapter 4).

Indeed, it is helpful to look at this from another angle and to view the therapeutic training of mental health practitioner researchers and the lived experience of mental health service user researchers as providing a basis from which the relationship issues within the data collection can be reflected upon, understood and managed. Coyle and Wright (1996) have suggested that an ability to use basic counselling skills is essential in facilitating data collection in connection with 'sensitive' topics and it has been commented upon that 'all too often' in-depth interviews have been conducted by researchers without interview training that considers how to build and maintain appropriate rapport (Thompson & Russo, in press). Coyle and Wright (1996) do not suggest – nor do we – that qualitative researchers need to be therapists or counsellors, rather that researchers have experiential training in how to build rapport and how to manage affect (see also Coyle, 1998).

Most mental health practitioners will be well experienced in their ability to deal with emotional charged situations and be able to stay with participants at the conclusion of an interview so as to contain these reactions and recommend further support if needed. Arguably, service user researchers will also have gained experience of maintaining rapport and staying with emotionally charged topics within a relational context. In any event, interview training that involves role-play and draws upon basic counselling skills (such as paraphrasing, summarizing, empathy, genuineness and unconditional positive regard) should be routinely provided to novice researchers and the beneficial similarities between practice, service user experience and research could be made more explicit by seasoned researchers.

Power and Politics

Research does not occur in a vacuum but is typically driven by an agenda, which may actively seek to guide or change mental health policy. Clearly, in such a situation power and politics will play a part and researchers should be reflexive in relation to considering the role their own ambitions may have on the research process.

Researchers taking a feminist position have long advocated that researchers engage in some degree of reciprocity so as to reduce power imbalances and also to build rapport (Oakley, 1981). It may be appropriate in some circumstances to share personal information to allow the participant to make an informed choice about whether or not to participate. For example, whilst a would-be participant might be reassured about the boundaries of confidentiality, their decision to participate might be affected by the knowledge that the interviewer (or other members of the research team) have roles that may bring them into contact with the participant again in the future.

Clearly, it is not possible to remove all power imbalance in research (whether led by practitioners or service user researchers) and all researchers should consider the influence that power imbalances might have and attempt to minimize these. One tactic is to explore specifically what the potential power imbalances might be early on and to do this in conjunction with members of the potential participant community.

Future Directions, Concluding Comments and Some 'Practical Guidelines'

We hope this chapter has raised awareness of some of the subtle ethical issues and dilemmas that can be encountered in conducting qualitative research in the mental health field (e.g., in negotiating whether to continue to pursue a particular area of discussion when a participant is clearly upset).

Whilst our varied professional ethical guidelines interpret ethical principles for use within the specific mental health disciplines and set basic benchmarks of good practice, they do not offer 'solutions' to specific ethical dilemmas in the field. Interestingly, with the move towards greater interprofessional working there has been discussion of how social and health care professionals can develop a greater sense of shared ethical practice and there is also a need for greater involvement of the public in the development of shared codes of practice (see Banks, 2009; Banks et al., 2010).

The ability to be self-aware and to be able to reflect in relation to ethical dilemmas is a core competency of most mental health practitioners and we have described here how this skill should be developed to negotiate ethical dilemmas. We are not alone in suggesting that ethical issues are best addressed by open ongoing reflexive thought (see for example Clarke's, 2006, personal account in relation to nursing research and Davison's, 2004, account of social work research). Such a reflexive process may involve individual reflexivity, supervision and, importantly, involvement with the particular research population associated with any given study.

Despite the limitations of simple sets of guidelines we nevertheless thought it would be helpful to summarize some of the themes discussed in this chapter by creating a set of practical recommendations for facilitating ethical research practice of mental health practitioners conducting qualitative research and this can be seen in Table 3.1.

Table 3.1 Recommendations for facilitating ethical research practice of mental health practitioners conducting qualitative research

---

Research planning stage – and throughout the project
- Consider user involvement at the earliest possible point in the research process and engage with individuals from the potential research population to consider the management of ethical issues
- Obtain supervision to ensure discussion of ongoing ethical issues, and provide opportunities for developing researcher reflexivity
- Use a reflective diary to encourage reflection on ethical issues and to outline decision-making processes
- Ensure all researchers have adequate awareness and/or training on ethical issues
- Ensure all researchers engaging with participants have training so as to be comfortable in collecting data in situations where people may exhibit emotional reactions

Recruitment phase
- Consider factors that may influence how voluntary participants' consent is, especially when there has been prior or current contact
- Ensure potential participants are aware of the role of researcher vs. the role of the practitioner, so as to avoid therapeutic expectation
- Facilitate informed consent by providing multiple opportunities for participants to gain information about the study
- Check out the potential participants' assumptions about research in advance, including perceived impact, dissemination and use

Data collection phase
- Discuss confidentiality and privacy in a tangible way. For example, participants could be shown examples of how the information they provide will appear and be used and by whom
- Facilitate understanding of dual roles. Clarify the role of the clinician vs. researcher so the participant is clear. For example, explaining that the research role is purely to listen to people's experiences and not to address difficulties or explore change. If the research follows an action research model, or is linked to an intervention, explain clearly what the limits of any interventions will be, and who will be responsible for them

---

(Continued)

Table 3.1   *(Continued)*

- Facilitate processual consent (the opportunity for participants to provide consent in an ongoing fashion)
- Empower the participant to have control in relation to terminating data collection without having to provide reason (this may be achieved, for example, by making it explicit that the participant can switch off recording equipment at any point without asking)
- Spend an appropriate amount of time with the participants to allow the above to happen and also for time to discuss the experience of participating afterwards in an informal fashion

Analysis phase
- Ensure interpretations are grounded in the participants' accounts from the research interview, and not from information obtained from other roles
- Consider with participants what it will be like for them to read or see the work in its completed form

Dissemination phase
- Provide feedback and disseminate in an accessible fashion and in a way that is useful to all stakeholders (i.e., participants, staff, organizations, charitable groups, fundholders)
- Gain participants views on participation in the study
- Enhance anonymity (unless negotiated otherwise) by guarding against the use of lengthy excerpts and the use of specific personal demographic details of participants

Source: Adapted from a forthcoming publication: Thompson, A. R., & Russo, K. (in press). Ethical dilemmas for clinical psychologists in conducting qualitative research. *Qualitative Research in Psychology.*

To conclude, we have discussed how it can be all too easy for practitioner researchers to fall into making value judgements, as to what constitutes 'sensitive' research and who might be described as 'vulnerable', and what the implications might be of such sensitivities and vulnerabilities. Active early involvement with service users or members of the research population can assist in ensuring a qualitative study achieves the best ethical outcome. With this in mind, we wish to end the chapter with a call for greater engagement between service users, potential research participants and researchers in considering ethical issues from the earliest possible point in the research process and to do this in line with the advice laid out in the next chapter and with reference to the organizations listed in the further reading and useful websites box.

References

Adamis, D., Martin, F., Treloar, A. & Macdonald, D. (2005). Capacity, consent, and selection bias in a study of delirium. *Journal of Medical Ethics, 31*, 137–143.

Allmark, P., Boote, J., Chambers, E., Clarke, A., McDonnell, A., Thompson, A.R., *et al.* (2009). Ethical issues in the use of in-depth interviews: Literature review and discussion. *Research Ethics Review, 5*, 48–54.

American Psychological Association. (2010). *Ethical principles of psychologists and code of conduct (amended).* Washington, DC: APA.

Banks, S. (2009). From professional ethics to ethics in professional life: Implications for learning, teaching and study'. *Ethics and Social Welfare, 3*, 55–63.

Banks, S., Allmark, P., Barnes, M., Barr, H., Bryant, L., Cowburn, M., *et al.* (2010). Interprofessional ethics: A developing field? Notes from the Ethics and Social Welfare Conference, Sheffield, UK, May 2010. *Ethics and Social Welfare, 4*, 3. First published on: 29 October 2010 (iFirst) DOI: 10.1080/17496535.2010.516116.

Beauchamp, T.L. & Childress, J.F. (2001). *Principles of biomedical ethics* (5th edn). New York: Oxford University Press.

Brinkmann, S. & Kvale, S. (2008). Ethics in qualitative psychological research. In C. Willig & W. Stainton-Rogers (Eds.) *The Sage handbook of qualitative research in psychology.* 263–279). London: Sage.

Bristol Royal Infirmary Inquiry. (2001). *The Report of the Public Inquiry into children's heart surgery at the Bristol Royal Infirmary 1984–1995: Learning from Bristol.* London: The Stationary Office Limited.

British Association of Social Workers. (2002). *The code of ethics for social work.* Birmingham: British Association of Social Workers.

British Psychological Society. (2005). *Good practice guidelines for the conduct of psychological research within the NHS.* Leicester: British Psychological Society.

British Psychological Society. (2006). *Code of ethics and conduct.* Leicester: British Psychological Society.

British Psychological Society. (2007). *Conducting research on the internet: Guidelines for ethical practice in psychological research online.* Leicester: British Psychological Society.

British Psychological Society. (2008). *Conducting research with people not having the capacity to consent to their participation: A practical guide for researchers.* Leicester: British Psychological Society.

Bryant, L. & Beckett, J. (2006). The practicality and acceptability of an advocacy service in the emergency department for people attending following self-harm. Retrieved 14 September 2010, from University of Leeds, Leeds Institute of Health Sciences, web site http://www.leeds.ac.uk/lihs/psychiatry/staff/beckett_j.htm.

Carrick, R. (2006). Service user's ethical priorities for psychological research. Doctoral thesis, University of Plymouth, Plymouth, UK.

Clark, C.C., Scott, E.A., Boydell, K.M. & Goering, P. (1999). Effects of client interviewers on client-reported satisfaction with mental health services. *Psychiatric Services, 50*, 961–963.

Clarke, A. (2006). Qualitative interviewing: encountering ethical issues and challenges. *Nurse Researcher, 13*, 19–29.

Coyle, A. (1998). Qualitative research in counselling psychology: Using the counselling interview as a research instrument. In P. Clarkson (Ed.) *Counselling psychology: Integrating theory, research and supervised practice* (pp. 56–73). London: Routledge.

Coyle, A. & Wright, C. (1996). Using the counselling interview to collect research data on sensitive topics. *Journal of Health Psychology, 1*, 431–440.

Critical Psychiatry Website. Critical Psychiatry Webpage. Retrieved 24 September 2010 from http://www.uea.ac.uk/~wp276/psychiatryanti.htm.

Davison, J. (2004). Dilemmas in research: issues of vulnerability and disempowerment for the social worker/researcher. *Journal of Social Work Practice, 18*, 379–393.

Department of Health. (1991). *Local research ethics committees.* London: Department of Health.

Department of Health. (2005). Research governance framework for Health and Social care (2nd edn). Retrieved 30 June 2009 from http://www.dh.gov.uk/en/Publicationsandstatistics/Publications/PublicationsPolicyAndGuidance/DH_4008777.

Department of Health. (2007). *Best research for best health: A new national health research strategy*. Retrieved 30 June 2009 from http://www.dh.gov.uk/en/Publicationsandstatistics/Publications/PublicationsPolicyAndGuidance/Browsable/DH_4127225.

Donnison, J., Thompson, A.R. & Turpin, G. (2009). A qualitative study of the conceptual models employed by community mental health team staff. *International Journal of Mental Health Nursing, 18*, 310–317.

Forbat, L. & Henderson, J. (2003). "Stuck in the middle with you": the ethics and process of qualitative research with two people in an intimate relationship. *Qualitative Health Research, 13*, 1453–1462.

Fossey, E., Epstein, M., Findlay, R., Plant, G. & Harvey, C. (2002). Creating a positive experience of research for people with psychiatric disabilities by sharing feedback. *Psychiatric Rehabilitation Journal, 25*, 369–378.

Francis, R.D. (2009). *Ethics for psychologists* (2nd edn). Oxford: BPS Blackwell.

Gleeson, K. & Mortimore, C. (2010). The process model for research supervision on the Bristol course. *Clinical Psychology Forum, 213*, 29–33.

Goodacre, S.W. (2010). Falling research in the NHS: Abolish new research governance infrastructure. *British Medical Journal, 340*, c3449.

Graham, J., Grewal, I. & Lewis, J. (2007). *Ethics in social research: The views of research participants*. NatCen: London.

Graham, J., Lewis J. & Nicolaas, G. (2006). *A review of literature on empirical studies of ethical requirements and research participation*. ESRC/NatCen: London.

Haggerty, K.D. (2004). Ethics creep: Governing social science research in the name of ethics. *Qualitative Sociology, 27*, 391–414.

Health Professions Council. (2008). *Standard of conduct, performance and ethics* (2nd edn). Retrieved 24 September 2010 from http://www.hpc-uk.org/publications/index.asp?id=38.

Holland, K. (2007). The epistemological bias of ethics review: Constraining mental health research. *Qualitative Inquiry, 13*, 895–913.

INVOLVE. (2004) Ethics review in social care research: Option appraisal and guidelines by Jan Pahl: A response from INVOLVE. Retrieved 7 September 2010 from http://www.invo.org.uk/search.asp.

Jenkins, R. (2008). What do we mean by vulnerable? Presentation retrieved 9 September 2010 from University of Sheffield, Research Ethics Pages website: http://www.shef.ac.uk/ris/gov_ethics_grp/ethics/vulnerable-.html.

Liamputtong, P. (2007). *Researching the vulnerable: A guide to sensitive research methods*. London: Sage.

National Research Ethics Service. (2009). Information sheets and consent forms: Guidance for researchers and reviewers. Retrieved 14 September 2010 from http://www.nres.npsa.nhs.uk/applications/guidance/consent-guidance-and-forms/?esctl1431725_entryid62=67013.

National Research Ethics Service and INVOLVE. (2009). Statement: Patient and public involvement in research and research ethics committee review. Retrieved 7 September 2010 from http://www.invo.org.uk/search.asp.

Nursing and Midwifery Council. (2010). The code: Standards of conduct, performance and ethics for nurses and midwives. Retrieved 24 September 2010 from http://www.nmc-uk.org/,

Oakley, A. (1981). Interviewing women: a contradiction in terms. In H. Roberts (Ed.) *Doing feminist research* (pp. 30–61). London: Routledge.

Rosenblatt, P.C. (1995). Ethics of qualitative interviewing with grieving families. *Death Studies, 19*, 139–155.

Royal Liverpool Children's Inquiry. (2001). *Royal Liverpool Children's Inquiry Report.* London: The Stationary Office Limited.

Ruzek, J. & Zatzick, D. (2000). Ethical considerations in research participation among acutely injured trauma survivors: An empirical investigation. *General Hospital Psychiatry, 22*, 27–36.

Scott, D., Valery, P., Boyle, F. & Bain, C. (2002). Does research into sensitive areas do harm? Experiences of research participation after a child's diagnosis with Ewing's sarcoma. *Medical Journal of Australia, 177*, 507–510.

Small, R. (2001). Codes are not enough: What philosophy can contribute to the ethics of educational research. *Journal of Philosophy of Education, 35*, 387–406.

Sweeney, A., Beresford, P., Faulkner, A., Nettle, M. & Rose, D. (2009). *This is survivor research.* Ross-on-Wye: PCCS Books.

Thompson, A.R. & Russo, K. (in press). Ethical dilemmas for clinical psychologists in conducting qualitative research. *Qualitative Research in Psychology.*

Wolfensberger, W. (1972). *The principles of normalisation in human services.* Toronto: National Institute on Mental Retardation.

World Medical Association. (2002). *'Declaration of Helsinki' ethical principles for medical research involving human subjects.* Washington: World Medical Association.

Further reading and useful websites

National Research Ethics Service (NRES): www.nres.npsa.nhs.uk. This is the website for research ethics in the NHS and contains useful information on all aspects of NHS ethical procedures. For example, detailed information is provided about designing consent and information forms.

Research Ethics Guidebook. A resource for social scientists: www.ethicsguidebook.ac.uk. This helpful site sponsored by the Economic and Social Research Council (ESRC) provides additional information in considering ethical issues at all stages of the research process

Social Care Research Ethics Committee: www.screc.org.uk. This website provides information about applying for research ethics review, when conducting research in social service and other community settings and who to contact for further help

Wallcraft, J., Amering, M. & Schrank, B. (2009). *Handbook of service user involvement in mental health research.* Oxford: Wiley-Blackwell.

4

Participation and Service User Involvement

Alison Faulkner

Traditionally, service users have been the subjects of research carried out by others and have not had any part to play in the research process, far less an equal part. This chapter outlines the origins and growth of survivor research and its role in the user/survivor movement, alongside the increasing involvement of service users in mental health research more generally; the relevant policy framework underpinning this; and some principles and resources for good practice in collaborative research. The author is a mental health service user[1] and researcher by background, and has worked on a range of research projects, both user-led/user-controlled and collaborative in nature.

There is a distinction to be made between survivor research, or user-controlled research, and user involvement in research (the latter often referred to as collaborative research). It may help to imagine a continuum with survivor research at one end and consultation at the other (see below). In the middle we will find many variations on the theme of 'user involvement' or collaborative research.

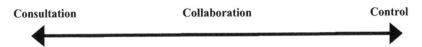

| Consultation | Collaboration | Control |

One of the issues fought over in the middle of this continuum is that of power. According to Turner and Beresford (2005), user involvement in research is seen to 'embody inequalities of power which work to the disadvantage of service users' (p. vi).

---

[1] 'Service user' is a term frequently used to refer to people who are diagnosed with a (usually long-term) mental health problem and are receiving or using services. Many people prefer the term 'survivor' because it states a political position of surviving the sometimes damaging and disempowering effects of services as well as surviving mental illness or distress.

Qualitative Research Methods in Mental Health and Psychotherapy: A Guide for Students and Practitioners, First Edition.
Edited by D. Harper and A.R. Thompson.
© 2012 John Wiley & Sons, Ltd. Published 2012 by John Wiley & Sons, Ltd.

History and Origins

The origins of survivor research lie within the development of the user/survivor move-ment, which can be traced back to evidence of dissatisfaction with mental health services voiced in the nineteenth century. It is generally agreed that it was in the mid 1980s that voices of protest became more recognizably organized as a user or survivor move-ment. Initially, the formation of hospital-based patients' councils and a proliferation of user-led self-help and advocacy groups developed alongside the formation of more formally organized networks such as Survivors Speak Out, the Hearing Voices Net-work and the UK Advocacy Network. Other contemporaneous developments included campaigns for women-only services and advocacy, and against the use of electrocon-vulsive therapy (ECT). The history of these initiatives is well documented by Campbell (1999, 2006).

Over the years, some prominent service user/survivor activists have made research their business, shaping and directing it towards being a useful and empowering tool for the service user/survivor movement. Many service users began to see the need to create their own knowledge which meant beginning to ask questions of each other, of groups and mailing lists in a systematic manner, as well as in some instances finding out about complex issues using more formal research methods.

At least one of the reasons for this lies in the desire (or need, even) for users or survivors of mental health services to create their own knowledge. For too long seen as the subjects of research, to be treated, measured and questioned by others, service users felt the need to challenge the power imbalance inherent in this form of research production and to take control of it: asking different questions, using different methods and finding out new things. Examples of survivor research began to emerge in the early 1990s in the alternative or 'grey' literature and in magazines such as *Asylum* (http://www.pccs-books.co.uk/section.php?xSec=284&xPage=1) and *Openmind* published by the UK charity Mind (Beeforth *et al.*, 1994; Cresswell, 1993; Wallcraft, 1993).

An excellent history of this development is given by Beresford and Wallcraft (1997). They make the link between survivor research and emancipatory disability research, which aims to empower or liberate service users through the research process. Research can emancipate people with disabilities/service users through challenging traditional research methods, adopting an inclusive and participatory approach to research and through describing people's individual or collective experience in their own terms. Survivor research (research by mental health service users/survivors) shares a common pathway with emancipatory research, in that it is controlled by mental health service users and has the aim of empowerment at its heart (Beresford & Wallcraft, 1997; Faulkner, 2004b). Similarly, there is a link with participatory research (and participatory action research) where the research question comes from the participating community and the aim is to bring about social change (Rose, 2004).

As Campbell (1999) points out, the UK service user/survivor movement has been dominated by association with service providers in the form of 'user involvement'. In this way, the energies of service users and survivors have been directed at changing and improving services rather more than developing user-led alternatives (Lindow, 1994).

> It has been both a blessing and a curse that service user/survivor action in the UK was engulfed so quickly in service-led enthusiasm for user involvement (Campbell, 1999, p. 207).

Indeed, national policy guidance has offered opportunities for groups and individuals to become involved in the mental health system in a variety of ways, from individual care through service evaluation to service delivery and planning and, of course, research. This sometimes symbiotic, sometimes parasitic relationship continues to this day.

The Policy Framework

Guidance from the UK Department of Health concerning the involvement of patients or service users in health research can be traced back at least as far as *Patient and Public Involvement in the NHS* (Department of Health, 1999). This document acknowledged the importance of service user involvement in many aspects of health service developments, including research, whilst *Research and Development for a First Class Service* (Department of Health, 2000) required Trusts holding NHS Research and Development (R&D) Support Funding to demonstrate evidence of involving service users in research activity.

The *Research Governance Framework for Health and Social Care* (Department of Health, 2005) states that '[r]elevant service users and carers or their representative groups should be involved wherever possible in the design, conduct, analysis and reporting of research' (2005, p. 8). The Framework comprises two areas of relevance to service users: a call for the active involvement of service users and carers at every stage of the research cycle; and a move towards greater openness about research undertaken by organizations. The organization INVOLVE (www.invo.org.uk) was established in 1995 as an advisory group to the Department of Health, with the aim of promoting public involvement in health, social care and public health research. For INVOLVE, public involvement can take place at any stage in the research cycle, from commissioning and funding research, through managing and design, fieldwork, analysis and interpretation of research and review and evaluation. Their core remit is to support public involvement in research in all its forms.

Service user involvement in research has increased incrementally in the last decade; many service users have chosen research as their core endeavour for involvement and change (Beresford & Wallcraft, 1997; Faulkner, 2004a; Lindow, 2001; Rose, 2003). Several units or departments dedicated to user involvement in research have become established in the last few years: for example, SURESearch at the University of Birmingham (www.suresearch.org.uk), and SURE (Service User Research Enterprise: http://www.iop.kcl.ac.uk/departments/?locator=300) at the Institute of Psychiatry in London (Box 4.1).

Box 4.1 Service User Research Enterprise, Institute of Psychiatry, London

The Service User Research Enterprise (SURE) aims to involve service users in a collaborative way throughout the whole research process: from design to data collection, through to data analysis and dissemination of results. Dr Diana Rose is co-director with Professor Til Wykes. Diana is a social scientist and a mental health service user; before joining the Institute of Psychiatry, she pioneered user-focused research at the then Sainsbury Centre for Mental Health.

SURE was launched in 2001 and is now one of the largest units within universities in Europe to employ people who have both research skills and first-hand experience of mental health services and treatments. The studies they have carried out include: Continuity of Care project, user involvement in change management, young people and primary care project and a systematic review of users' views of electroconvulsive therapy (ECT) which contributed to the NICE guidelines on ECT.

For more information: http://www.iop.kcl.ac.uk/departments/?locator=300

At a national level, the Mental Health Research Network (MHRN; www.mhrn.info) – a part of the UK National Institute for Health Research (NIHR; www.nihr.ac.uk) has a 'hub' dedicated to service user involvement in research adopted by the network. Originally termed the Service User Research Group, England or SURGE, this hub has now been re-formed as Service Users in Research (Box 4.2). The MHRN has published guidance for researchers about how to involve service users in research and is monitoring progress (Service User Research Group England, 2005).

Box 4.2 The National Institute for Health Research Mental Health Research Network: Service Users in Research

Service Users in Research plays an important part in making sure research across the Mental Health Research Network (MHRN) is valuable for and makes sense to service users. Service Users in Research supports service user input into the MHRN through service user involvement in local hub committees, research project teams and at a national level.

(Continued)

Box 4.2 (*Cont'd*)

Service User Forum for Research

The Forum is open to any service user or service user organization with an interest in mental health research. The Forum will offer the opportunity for people to share and discuss ideas concerning Service Users in Research and service user involvement in the MHRN. The first forum meeting took place in London in 2010 following the first MHRN PPI Conference. For more information contact:

Service Users in Research
Institute of Psychiatry
King's College London
PO Box 77
De Crespigny Park
London
SE5 8AF
E-mail: mhrnppi@kcl.ac.uk
Phone: 020 7848 0644
For more information: http://www.mhrn.info/index/ppi/SUR.html

Some voluntary organizations, such as the Mental Health Foundation (MHF) and the Centre for Mental Health (formerly the Sainsbury Centre for Mental Health), established programmes of work dedicated to 'user-led' research which recognized and supported the potential of service users to undertake their own research. The MHF funded an innovative project called Strategies for Living (Box 4.3).

Box 4.3 Strategies for Living

The Mental Health Foundation's Strategies for Living programme ran from 1997 to 2003. Funded by the National Lottery, the programme aimed 'to document and disseminate people's strategies for living with mental distress' through research as well as through networks, newsletters and publications.

The first phase consisted of a qualitative research project: 'Strategies for Living: *A report of user-led research into People's Strategies for Living with Mental Distress.* (Faulkner & Layzell, 2000). Six service users were trained and supported to undertake the interviews for the research. The project also supported six user-led

(Continued)

Box 4.3 (*Cont'd*)

research projects through funding, training and support (Nicholls, 2001). The second phase (2000–2003) supported 16 projects around the United Kingdom, all of which were initiated by local user groups or individuals (Nicholls *et al.*, 2003).

The programme was innovative in that it sought from the start to be entirely led by service users and to support user-led research, although based within a mental health charity. All of the team were people with direct experience of mental distress and/or of using mental health services.

The impact of the policy developments over the last two decades has been to introduce into a range of public funding streams the requirement for researchers to demonstrate in funding applications how service users will be involved in their research projects (e.g., the National Coordinating Centre for Health Technology Assessment programme, www.hta.ac.uk; and the NHS Service Delivery and Organization programme, www.sdo.nihr.ac.uk). It has also resulted in public involvement being on the agenda of the National Institute for Health Research (NIHR; www.nihr.ac.uk) and within the individual research networks including the MHRN.

One of the unfortunate consequences of these developments has been to dilute the nature and impact of the involvement; what may have started out as *service user* involvement with its roots in survivor research and emancipatory research, has now become *public* involvement, which can include many stakeholders in the research production. The terms of reference for INVOLVE (http://www.invo.org.uk/terms.asp, retrieved 5 September 2010) refer to 'the public'; this includes: consumers; patients and potential patients; people who use health and social services; informal (unpaid) carers and parents; members of the public who may be targeted by health promotion programmes; organizations that represent the public's interests; communities that are affected by health, public health or social care issues.

Whilst this may seem a logical development in many ways, it can mean that voluntary organizations or other agences operating on behalf of service users or patients may become involved in their stead. This does not represent quite the same challenge nor does it offer quite the same potential contribution to the research.

At this point, it is worth pointing out that, although this chapter mainly focuses on service user involvement in undertaking research, service users can be involved at any stage (or indeed all stages) of the research cycle. Service users are involved in commenting on research proposals for some funding bodies and may be involved in commissioning decisions or sit on research ethics committees on occasions. Some academic departments and some funding bodies may engage a group of service users as a reference group to consult about research ideas and applications. However, one of the least rewarding and least influential of roles is to be a single service user on a research advisory group, as this can be undertaken with the aim of ticking the 'user involvement box' but without thought given to how the individual can participate in the discussion in a meaningful way.

Research Methods

The methods themselves play a significant part in the development of survivor research. Many service users and survivors believe it is not enough simply to do the same research with different characters playing the parts. People have sought instead to use methods that will empower research participants, treat people with respect and listen to their stories rather than treating them as objects without their own contributions to offer to the research process. In the disability field, emancipatory research (underpinned by a social model of disability) pre-dated the developments in survivor research. Barnes and Mercer (1997) say that emancipatory research in the disability context should be enabling rather than disabling and that it should be 'reflexive' and self-critical. For the research to be reflexive, service user/survivor researchers need to examine honestly the ways in which their identity as researchers and as people with experience of using mental health services may have affected the research and the interpretations flowing from it.

For some people, qualitative research is inherently empowering in that it listens to and communicates the actual words of research participants. But, for service users and survivor researchers engaged in research, research needs to go further than that in order to achieve a shift in the balance of power. This means service users themselves being engaged in the research process, analysing and interpreting the voices of their peers and ensuring that the findings get back to the communities from which they arise with the aim of bringing about positive change in people's lives.

These developments have led to new topics being researched, the use of new methods and a change in the research process. The significance of research from the user/survivor perspective is that it can challenge current notions of evidence and promote the development of user-defined outcomes. It can formulate alternative understandings and find out what helps people who are currently dissatisfied with the existing services on offer. A key issue lies in knowing what questions to ask and in building the kind of trust that comes from speaking together as peers. As pointed out by Lindow (2001), research is never a neutral act and the research of mental health professionals is increasingly understood to have its own agendas and culture. Lindow finishes her chapter as follows:

> Research has its part to play in developing solidarity among psychiatric system survivors, and helping to raise the expectations of those who have been "educated" to live with an unacceptable quality of life. Survivor research can be a small but key part in the move to seize freedom within an oppressive and excluding society (Lindow, 2001, p. 145).

This approach to research often, but by no means exclusively, leads us to use qualitative research methods. One reason for this is the opportunity that some qualitative methods give for people to tell their stories and for those stories to be listened to, taken account of and reported for others to hear. The tendency for the majority of mental health professionals to focus their questions around specific symptoms and diagnoses (as dictated by the medical model) often means that people have little opportunity to tell their stories, and in doing so begin to make sense of their own experiences:

> I am tired of being talked about, treated as a statistic, pushed to the margins of human conversation. I want someone who will have time for me, someone who will listen to me, someone who has not already judged who I am or what I have to offer. I am waiting to be taken seriously (service user quoted in Nicholls and the Somerset Spirituality Project Research Team, 2002, p. 1).

Mainstream quantitative research, which regards the randomized controlled trial (RCT) as the gold standard, underpins the established understanding of 'evidence-based medicine'. It is one of the mainstays of the power held by, in this case, the psychiatric establishment. Consequently, the tendency for service user and survivor research to take a qualitative approach presents us with a dilemma because it is inherently less powerful in the research world because of the dominance of quantitative approaches. However, within this context, it should be noted that SURE (Box 4.1) has developed innovative and progressive ways of involving service users in large-scale quantitative research projects.

Although qualitative research does not have the status or the power to persuade of the RCT, it can offer us the opportunity to create our own knowledge without too many preconceived notions about what we are looking for. For some survivor researchers, this has also been a source of frustration, as we have not comprehensively developed our own theoretical approach. Still, much of the research undertaken in mental health that actively involves service users as research participants is directed at existing services and treatments rather than at survivor-directed initiatives. There is quite simply less funding available for user-controlled research or for user-controlled initiatives. Although service users are involved to some extent (e.g., in the NIHR) they do not have equal power to direct research priorities or policy developments.

Benefits of Service User Involvement

There is little actual 'evidence' concerning the benefits (or otherwise) of involving service users in research. A recent report commissioned by INVOLVE presents the results of a literature review to establish the evidence base for public involvement in research (Staley, 2009). One of their key recommendations is that researchers should document the levels and impact of public involvement in their research, and that journals should also encourage this in their guidelines.

Nevertheless, a number of researchers, service users and service user/survivor researchers have written about the benefits that they have seen or experienced. Service User Research Group England (2005) included a literature review which discussed the benefits of involving service users in mental health research. Several papers suggested that the service user perspective itself brought benefits with it. By offering insight into what it feels like to experience mental health problems, to use mental health services or to receive certain treatments, service users can help ensure that research is more relevant to clinical practice and the results more relevant to service users (Allam *et al.*, 2004; Goodare & Lockwood, 1999; Hanley *et al.*, 2003; Rose, 2003; Trivedi & Wykes, 2002).

Involvement at the design stage

A vital stage for service user involvement is when the research questions are being drafted or, in the case of quantitative research, when outcome measures are being selected. Allam *et al.* (2004) discuss the benefits of involving service users and carers in the design of relevant questions in qualitative reseasrch. Such benefits include the fact that questions are more grounded in real experience and in consequence are more meaningful and relevant than those developed by non-service user researchers. Trivedi and Wykes (2002) describe the negotiation needed to determine the outcome measures used in quantitative research because service users and clinicians may regard different outcomes and hence outcome measures to be important. This also highlights the importance of service users being involved at an early stage of project development in order to allow for enough time to agree on outcome measures relevant to both. Wykes (2003) develops this further, exploring the benefits of service user involvement to the research questions, outcome measures and the overall methods used.

Ramon (2000) contends that user involvement in the research process leads to the generation of new and more in-depth knowledge in the field of mental health. She also suggests it leads to researchers gaining a better understanding of the lives of service users and of lay perceptions of research as well as those of service users.

Recruitment

Several researchers refer to the way in which service users might assist in finding and providing access to potential participants, particularly members of marginalized groups (e.g., Fleischmann & Wigmore, 2000; Hanley *et al.*, 2003). Researchers often find it difficult to access people from marginalized communities, many of whom are reluctant to have research done 'to' or 'for' them. They are much more likely to work with researchers who want to collaborate with them on research that has been identified by the service user community as a priority, or with researchers who are willing to support them to undertake their own research.

Interviewing

Several researchers and service users report that, where service users are engaged as interviewers, they may obtain more open and honest responses from research participants (Allam *et al.*, 2004; Faulkner & Layzell, 2000; Polowycz *et al.*, 1993; Ramon, 2000; Rose, 2001). This is not a universal finding – for example, Clark *et al.* (1999) found little difference overall between the responses made to client as opposed to professional interviewers, although in the former, client or peer researchers were found to elicit more negative or critical responses. However, Gillard and Turner (2008), reporting on a project at the UK MHRN scientific conference, suggested that there were differences in the emphasis placed on issues followed up in qualitative interviews between service user and non-service user interviewers. The authors reported that service user interviewers were more likely to follow up issues relating to personal experience and feelings, whereas non-service user interviewers focused more on issues of procedure.

Analysis

Allam *et al.* (2004) suggest that the differences in the interpretation of responses between service users and carers (and potentially professionals) provide a strong justification for involving service users and carers at the analysis stage. They suggest that the validity of the findings can be improved by working together and coming to a joint agreement about the meaning of the data. Faulkner *et al.* (2008) also comment on the value of involving service users throughout the research, including the analysis stage in a complex qualitative research project (Box 4.4).

Box 4.4 Learning the Lessons: Evaluation of Community Services for People with a Diagnosis of Personality Disorder

This research study was a collaboration between the Mental Health Foundation, Imperial College London, University College London, the Institute of Psychiatry and the University of Liverpool. The study comprised four research modules, one of which was a user-led evaluation of the services undertaken by the Mental Health Foundation. A team of service user interviewers and researchers based at MHF evaluated service quality from the perspective of service users and carers in contact with the 11 services under evaluation.

The user-led module involved and included service users and carers throughout the project: as representatives on the steering group and project advisory group and as researchers conducting interviews and analysing the data. The research has been written up in a number of ways (e.g., Crawford *et al.*, 2007; Faulkner *et al.*, 2008; Price *et al.*, 2009).

Dissemination

Several researchers and service users report the benefits of service user involvement at the dissemination stage of research (e.g., Telford *et al.*, 2002). Hanley *et al.* (2003) report that voluntary organizations may assist in dissemination by carrying summaries of research in user-friendly language in their newsletters and magazines. Trivedi and Wykes (2002) also suggest publishing research on websites. This has been demonstrated by research carried out under the umbrella of the Mental Health Foundation's Strategies for Living project and the Sainsbury Centre's User Focused Monitoring projects (Rose et al., 1998).

Challenges of Service User Involvement

There are a number of challenges involved, some of which are practical, some philosophical and some interpersonal. Some of these issues are not so much challenges as indicators of need; for example, there is a need to provide training and support if the involvement of service users in research is to succeed.

There is some anecdotal evidence to suggest that the greatest difficulties experienced by service users are attitudinal (see also Faulkner, 2004b). At the basis of this are issues of power and control, and a belief that people who have mental health problems cannot be expected to understand or contribute to what is seen as a fundamentally rational process. Some researchers fear that involving service users will have a negative impact on the quality of research because they may have no professional research skills and because of a belief that they may be biased or lack objectivity.

Some researchers may feel reluctant to share control or be anxious about doing so for fear of losing their own power or status. From the service user point of view, the power issue is central. Service users usually come to the table with less power over the research process or the way in which the research is conducted. Explicitly sharing power with service users is likely to establish trust and lead to a more productive collaboration (for an example of collaborative research see Box 4.4).

Involving service users in research brings with it the need for additional resources in terms of money and time; this can be offputting to researchers and is often not built in to project proposals to ensure that the resources are there from the start. Although it is important not to make assumptions, some service users will have no research experience and some may have few educational qualifications. Like anyone new to research, they are likely to need training and this has implications for resources. There are a number of publications available that offer guidance on training and support for involvement (e.g., Faulkner, 2004a,b; INVOLVE, 2007; Nicholls et al., 2003; Sweeney et al., 2008).

People with mental health problems may need more support than other members of a research team. Faulkner (2004b) distinguishes between three different kinds of support: practical or administrative support; emotional support; and supervisory support. Mechanisms for support can be built into a project to the benefit of everyone involved. Indeed, many junior researchers embark on their careers with little support or training. As with training, an assessment of need should take place and there should not be a blanket assumption that everyone has the same support needs.

One of the implications of collaborative research is a need for compromise and a willingness to carry out research in a different way. Researchers need to be flexible and make both research and management procedures explicit and accessible. Service users may have good ideas about how to do the research (e.g., knowing how or when to access service user participants on an inpatient ward; good practice in conducting an interview with someone in distress). It is essential that researchers are open-minded and do not assume that they know best; the best research is likely to learn from the expertise of both.

Many of these issues might have an impact on conventional project management responsibilities. In order to avoid a project falling behind schedule or needing more resources because someone has become ill or needs additional support, research managers need to take these factors into account when planning the study. However, with all of these challenges in mind, the benefits are worth it. Box 4.5 gives an outline of good practice for collaborative research.

Box 4.5 Good Practice in Collaborative Research

1 Underlying Principles

The available work on survivor research and user involvement highlights the value of maintaining principles of, for example: clarity and transparency; empowerment; access and accessibility; clarity of identity; commitment to change; respect; and equal opportunities (for further explanation see Faulkner, 2004a).

2 Planning and Design

Think about the following issues at the planning stage:

- How to involve service users from the start
- Budget for involvement: to include payment of expenses and fees, support and training options
- Plan how you will be providing support
- Planning for flexibility – being open to negotiation, remaining flexible about people's involvement

3 Training

Training needs to enable service users to take part on an equal basis. It is good practice to train service users and non-service user researchers together so that everyone learns together and from each other. Training can include: introduction to research; ethical issues; interviewing skills (with role-play); how to ask questions; and so on (Faulkner, 2004a; Nicholls, 2001; Nicholls et al., 2003).

4 Support and Supervision

It is important to recognize the potential needs of service users for support as well as for supervision. Some people may need emotional support for undertaking

(Continued)

Box 4.5 (*Cont'd*)

the work, particularly if it covers ground familiar to their own experience; some people may need administrative support, particularly if they have not worked in an office environment before (Faulkner, 2004a).

5 Analysis and Interpretation

Analysis and interpretation of results is another key phase of the research that can benefit from service user involvement. Training in analysis can be offered to some; others may prefer to be involved in discussing the findings and offering interpretation from a service user perspective.

6 Dissemination and Implementation

Involving service users in dissemination may help not only in enabling access to service user groups and networks, but also in assisting with making the findings accessible to a service user audience whether in written form or speaking at conferences and so on.

Conclusions

Despite the many developments outlined in this chapter, service user involvement in mental health research is not comprehensive. As service users, we do not have an equal place at the table where the decisions are made. There are a number of reasons for this, as we have seen in this chapter, most of which take us back to the fundamental power imbalance. In a world dominated by rationality and order, people who are seen as 'defined by our unreason or irrationality, closeness to brute nature and overwhelmed by our emotions' (Rose, 2004, p. 28) are unlikely to hold much power.

Nevertheless, some would argue that it is our right to be involved in publicly funded research: to have a say in what is researched and in how it is carried out (see Faulkner & Thomas, 2002; Telford & Faulkner, 2004). If research in the twenty-first century is to be relevant, practicable and useful to the furthering of health and social care developments, then surely it has to involve the people who are at the receiving end of health and social care provision.

References

Allam, S., Blyth, S., Fraser, A., Hodgson, S., Howes, J., Repper, J., *et al.* (2004). Our experience of collaborative research: Service users, carers and researchers work together to evaluate an assertive outreach service. *Journal of Psychiatric and Mental Health Nursing, 11,* 368–373.

Barnes, C. & Mercer, G. (Eds.) (1997). *Doing disability research.* Leeds: Disability Press.

Beeforth, M., Conlan, E. & Graley, R. (1994). *Have we got views for you: User evaluation of case management.* London: Sainsbury Centre for Mental Health.

Beresford, P. & Wallcraft, J. (1997). Psychiatric system survivors and emancipatory research: Issues, overlaps and differences. In C. Barnes & G. Mercer (Eds.) *Doing disability research.* Leeds: Disability Press.

Campbell, P. (1999). The service user/survivor movement, in C. Newnes, G. Holmes & C. Dunn (Eds.)*This is madness: A critical look at psychiatry and the future of mental health services.* Ross-on-Wye: PCCS Books.

Campbell, P. (2006). *Some things you should know about user/survivor action.* A Mind resource pack. London: Mind.

Clark C.C., Scott, E.A., Boydell, K.M. & Goering, P. (1999). Effects of client interviewers on client-reported satisfaction with mental health services. *Psychiatric Services, 50,* 961–963.

Crawford, M., Rutter, D., Price, K., Weaver, T., Josson, M., Tyrer, P., *et al.* (2007). *Learning the lessons: A multi-method evaluation of dedicated community-based services for people with personality disorder.* London: National Coordinating Centre for NHS Service Delivery and Organization R&D.

Cresswell, J. (1993). Users' report on psychiatric services, *Asylum, 23,* 7.

Department of Health. (1999). *Patient and public involvement in the new NHS.* London: Department of Health.

Department of Health. (2000). *Research and development for a first class service.* London: Department of Health.

Department of Health. (2005). *Research governance framework for health and social care* (2nd edn). London: Department of Health.

Faulkner, A. (2004a). The ethics of survivor research: Guidelines for the ethical conduct of research carried out by mental health service users and survivors. Bristol: Policy Press on behalf of the Joseph Rowntree Foundation. Retrieved 5 September 2010 from http://www.jrf.org.uk/publications/ethics-survivor-research-guidelines-ethical-conduct-research-carried-out-mental-health-.

Faulkner, A. (2004b). *Capturing the experiences of those involved in the TRUE Project: A story of colliding worlds.* Eastleigh: INVOLVE. (Also available at www.invo.org.uk.)

Faulkner, A., Gillespie, S., Imlack, S., Dhillon, K. & Crawford, M. (2008). Learning the lessons together. *Mental Health Today, 8* (February), 24–26.

Faulkner, A. & Layzell, S. (2000). *Strategies for living: A report of user-led research into people's strategies for living with mental distress.* London: Mental Health Foundation.

Faulkner, A. & Thomas, P. (2002). User-led research and evidence based medicine. *British Journal of Psychiatry, 180,* 1–3.

Fleischmann, P. & Wigmore, J. (2000). *Nowhere else to go: Increasing choice and control within supported housing for homeless people with mental health problems.* London: Single Homeless Project.

Gillard, S. & Turner, K. (2008). Does who we are make a difference to the research that we do? Paper presented at UK Mental Health Research Network National Scientific Conference, Royal College of Physicians, London, 26–29 March.

Goodare, H. & Lockwood, S. (1999). Involving patients in clinical research. *British Medical Journal, 319,* 724–725.

Hanley, B., Bradburn, J., Barnes, M., Evans, C., Goodare, H., Kelson, M., *et al.* (2003). In: R. Steel (Ed.) *Involving the public in NHS, public health, and social care research: Briefing notes for researchers* (2nd edn). Eastleigh: INVOLVE. (Available at www.invo.org.uk.)

INVOLVE. (2007). *Public information pack.* Eastleigh: INVOLVE (Also available at www.invo.org.uk.)

Lindow, V. (1994). *Self-help alternatives to mental health services.* London: MIND.

Lindow, V. (2001). Survivor research. In C. Newnes, G. Holmes & C. Dunn (Eds.) *This is madness: A critical look at psychiatry and the future of mental health services.* Ross-on-Wye: PCCS Books.

Nicholls, V. (2001). *Doing research ourselves.* London: Mental Health Foundation.

Nicholls, V. & Somerset Spirituality Project Research Team. (2002). *Taken seriously: The Somerset Spirituality Project.* London: Mental Health Foundation.

Nicholls, V., Wright, S., Waters, R. & Wells, S. (2003). *Surviving user-led research: Reflections on supporting user-led research projects.* London: Mental Health Foundation.

Polowycz, D., Brutus, M., Orvietto, B.S., Vidal, J. & Cipriana, D. (1993). Comparison of patient and staff surveys of consumer satisfaction. *Hospital and Community Psychiatry, 44,* 589–691.

Price, K., Gillespie, S., Rutter, D., Dhillon, K., Gibson, S., Faulkner, A., *et al.* (2009). Dedicated personality disorder services: A qualitative analysis of service structure and treatment process. *Journal of Mental Health, 18,* 467–475.

Ramon, S. (2000). Participative mental health research: Users and professional researchers working together. *Mental Health Care, 3,* 224–228.

Rose, D. (2001). *Users' voices: The perspectives of mental health service users on community and hospital care.* London: Sainsbury Centre for Mental Health.

Rose, D. (2003). Collaborative research between users and professionals: Peaks and pitfalls. *Psychiatric Bulletin, 27,* 404–406.

Rose, D. (2004). Telling different stories: User involvement in mental health research. *Research Policy and Planning, 22* (2), 23–30.

Rose, D., Ford, R., Lindley, P., Gawith, L. & the KCW Mental Health Monitoring Users' Group. (1998). *In our experience: User focused monitoring of mental health services in Kensington & Chelsea and Westminster Health Authority.* London: Sainsbury Centre for Mental Health.

Service User Research Group England. (2005). *Guidance for good practice: Service user involvement in the UK Mental Health Research Network.* London: UK MHRN.

Staley, K. (2009). *Exploring impact: Public involvement in NHS, public health and social care research.* Eastleigh: INVOLVE.

Sweeney, A., Beresford, P., Faulkner, A., Nettle, M. & Rose D. (Eds.) (2008). *This is survivor research.* Ross-on-Wye: PCCS Books.

Telford, R., Beverley, C.A., Cooper, C.L. & Boote, J.D. (2002). Consumer involvement in health research: Fact or fiction? *British Journal of Clinical Governance, 7,* 92–103.

Telford, R. & Faulkner, A. (2004). Learning about user involvement in mental health research. *Journal of Mental Health, 13,* 549–559.

Trivedi, P. & Wykes, T. (2002). From passive subjects to equal partners. *British Journal of Psychiatry, 181,* 468–472.

Turner, M. & Beresford, P. (2005). *Contributing on equal terms: Service user involvement and the benefits system.* London: Social Care Institute for Excellence.

Wallcraft, J. (1993). Self-advocacy in 1992, *Openmind, 61,* 7.

Wykes, T. (2003). Blue skies in the *Journal of Mental Health*: Consumers in research. *Journal of Mental Health, 12,* 1–6.

Further reading and useful website

Staley, K. (2009) *Exploring impact: Public involvement in NHS, public health and social care research*. Eastleigh: INVOLVE.

Sweeney, A., Beresford, P., Faulkner, A., Nettle, M. & Rose D. (Eds.) (2008). *This is survivor research*. Ross-on-Wye: PCCS Books.

Wallcraft, J., Schrank, B. & Amering, M. (Eds.) (2009). *Handbook of service user involvement in mental health research*. Chichester: Wiley-Blackwell.

See also the INVOLVE website www.invo.org.uk for a range of downloadable publications concerning public involvement in research.

5

Qualitative Data Collection: Asking the Right Questions

Hannah Frith and Kate Gleeson

What Data Collection Method Should I Use?

Qualitative research undertaken by therapists and mental health practitioners is often fraught with problems because we usually want to address problems that arise in practice, rather than questions that arise out of extensive appraisal of a literature. The ostensible purpose of research may be to make a contribution to knowledge, but we typically want to make a contribution to practice, albeit evidence-based practice. This often means trying to understand the experience of an under-researched group or defining a new construct or territory within a neglected topic area. It is sometimes hard to link the questions that arise in clinical contexts to well-established bodies of knowledge. As a result, inexperienced qualitative researchers frequently engage in small-scale exploratory projects, with often ill-defined but clinically important questions. Fortunately, it is not the task of this chapter to consider the problems of how to analyse data from exploratory studies in a way that connects to existing literature and makes sense of the findings well enough to use in practice. These issues are substantively dealt with throughout the book (most notably in Chapters 2 and 16).

Nonetheless, the exploratory study with a relatively open question, while problematic, is full of intriguing possibilities and often gives rise to the most interesting and creative use of data collection devices. Although novice researchers frequently assume that interviews are the only or 'best' method of data collection, we aim to give a flavour of the infinite variety of techniques available, and the ways in which these can be adapted to meet the needs of particular projects. Trying to address the vast range of methods in a single chapter would mean that we would only be able to discuss each in a very superficial way. Instead, we want to alert the reader to the range of possibilities, and

Qualitative Research Methods in Mental Health and Psychotherapy: A Guide for Students and Practitioners, First Edition.
Edited by D. Harper and A.R. Thompson.
© 2012 John Wiley & Sons, Ltd. Published 2012 by John Wiley & Sons, Ltd.

to help you think about the issues that you will need to address when trying to decide which method to adopt.

We have structured the chapter around a set of questions which will allow us to address the themes of ethics, power, reflexivity, service user involvement, pragmatics and epistemology, as well as discussing and giving examples of how a wide range of data collection methods (including observation ethnography, naturally occurring conversation, individual interviews, group interviews, sampling of existing documentation, visual techniques and diaries) intersect with these issues. Of course, we cannot discuss all of these methods and issues simultaneously so we have to artificially separate them out in order to examine and explain them. In doing this we necessarily simplify, often flipping between hiding differences between methods and approaches, or exaggerating them in order to make a point clear. We provide a summary table, which is an attempt to clarify and to plug gaps where not every issue is discussed in relation to each type of data collection.

It is important to emphasize from the outset that there is no formula that produces good research (see Chapter 16). Research design is a creative and iterative process. Some crucial decisions need to be made right from the beginning if the research project is to be productive (see Chapters 3 and 7), but many smaller questions (such as the specific questions to ask in an interview, how many different data collection events or how many data need to be collected) will not be answered until the data collection is underway. Therefore, designs grow over time, developing as a function of the growing body of knowledge and the increasing skill and confidence of the researcher. This is perhaps why reflexivity is the crucial tool of the qualitative researcher.

Just as there is no magic formula for research design, it is also the case that there is no 'right' way to implement a particular qualitative method. While some try to set up 'rule books' to channel researchers towards the 'correct' implementation of a particular method, we believe that attempts to keep a rigid set of steps in place often fail for the same reason that parenting manuals fail – because the children have not read them! Our participants have not read the book and stubbornly refuse to follow the rules. No method should be fixed and inflexible, and most can be adapted, modified and altered to fit the particular needs of any research situation. Indeed, the most successful methodologies are those that allow for development and creativity.

It is this adaptability that enables the researcher to 'fit' the method to their epistemology, to their research question, to their own skills, experience and ways of being in the world, to their participants and to the kinds of knowledge that they aim to produce. It is this adaptability that allows us to generate innovative, insightful and useful knowledge. Therefore, the key starting point must be, what kind of knowledge is the researcher trying to produce?

Does the Data Collection Method Allow Me to Answer my Research Question?

This may sound like an obvious or easy question, but in our experience it is deceptively so. Too often research questions are vague or poorly defined, or methods are adopted which are not suitable for addressing the question posed. Different methods of data collection structure the process of gathering data and the sort of knowledge that is generated in particular ways – even when they appear to be doing a similar job. For example, diaries are particularly useful for gathering information about the day-to-day experiences of participants, and allow researchers to see these activities within the context of other aspects of daily life. This method depends on participants accurately recording their lives, being attuned to what the researcher might want to know and being inclined to report this. Therefore, diaries can produce knowledge about day-to-day activities and also the meaning that this holds for participants. Alternatively, recordings of naturalistic conversations also allow access to everyday life and ordinary worlds, but do not require the participant to filter and package the information for the researcher. However, the knowledge produced is a 'snapshot' of these activities and focuses only on what is said. Similarly, observation allows access to everyday experience which the researcher observes for themselves but they may not have access the meaning of these activities for participants. Therefore, different methods structure the experience of the researcher and the research participant (which we return to later), and each produce different knowledge whilst focusing ostensibly on the same question of everyday experience (for a fully discussion of choosing methods more generally see Chapter 7).

Moving continuously between the research question and the method of data collection allows for a more specific and detailed research question to emerge. Imagine that you want to examine the process of recovery from eating disorders. One way to research this question would be to conduct an ethnography of an inpatient eating disorders unit because you believe that an engaged period of observation and the opportunity to interview 'key informants' would avoid a 'snapshot' approach and would allow you to take seriously the idea that recovery is a process that unfolds over time. This decision would reflect a number of assumptions about the nature of recovery (as a medical event) and where recovery takes place (within medical settings). Such an approach would foreground clinical definitions of recovery and expertise perhaps at the expense of the lived experience of those recovering from eating disorders. This may lead you to reconsider the specificity of your question: How is recovery from eating disorders constructed by staff and patients in an inpatient eating disorders unit? Alternatively, you may decide that you would prefer to adopt a more client-centred approach to the issue of recovery and therefore you may reconsider the method and decide to conduct in-depth biographical interviews with women who are working towards recovery. You cannot ask a research question without discursively constructing 'objects' within the question. Each of the terms that we use (recovery, carer, female, psychosis) will be packed with meanings, which must be made explicit if we are to operationalize them in data collection. Considering what kinds of information a data collection method will produce, and the assumptions that underpin both the methods and the objects embedded in the research question, will enable you to clarify your research focus and ensure that the method you select will enable you to address your research question.

Does the Data Collection Technique Fit with the Epistemological Assumptions that Underlie the Research?

One of the most frustrating things about choosing a data collection technique is that it can appear to be a relatively neutral task. You pick up a recipe book of techniques, choose one that seems to allow you to gather the right shape and kind of data, and off you go. You start to compare what you are doing with other researchers and often find that you appear to be doing the same thing but by a different name and with vastly different implications, or you find that you are doing very different things but they claim to be using the same approach using the same steps. This confusion probably arises from the basic fact that there are only so many things you can do with qualitative data (i.e., most forms of analysis involve coding and categorizing the data in order to summarize and interpret it). The actions you take are more determined by the kind of participants you have and the kind of topic you are exploring than by the method you adopt. However, the most important thing about what you are doing, and the thing that will most affect the status of your data is your epistemological position – how you understand what you are doing. We will illustrate this by thinking about the interview as a popular data collection device used by researchers with a vast range of epistemological positions.

The standard research methods text tends to talk about interviews in terms of whether they are structured or unstructured. Although helpful in terms of thinking about the extent to which the interview schedule should be determined in advance, this provides no other clue about how to proceed. All interviews are structured, all social interactions are structured. One key difference between epistemological approaches to interviewing is to do with how the social structure of the interview is understood, and what the researcher thinks happens in an interview.

A traditional empirical approach to the interview, of the kind that Kinsey *et al.* (1948) undertook, assumes that the key to the interview is a well-designed and pre-tested interview schedule. This allows questions to be asked in an ideal order, with a consistency and reliability that ensures that any differences that appear in the talk of the interviewee are to do with the peculiarities of that interviewee. Issues of control, demand characteristics, validity and objectivity are key. The participant is the passive retainer of the data, and the interviewer has to skilfully press the right buttons in order to acquire it.

In contrast, when adopting a Interpretative Phenomenological Analysis (IPA, see also Chapter 8) approach we are interested in the individual and the particularities of their understanding, but we do not see them as passive actors in the drama. If we are going to really understand their point of view we cannot assume we know even what questions to ask to allow them to explain this to us. We have to negotiate our way into the topic to find a common ground of understanding. Therefore we begin with (very few) open questions, rather than a detailed interview schedule replete with prompts and probes. We know the territory we want to approach and have key areas to touch on, but we do not know the route that we will take to get there. The journey is as much determined by the interviewee as it is by the interviewer. There is no aspiration towards objectivity. The interview is understood as a reflexive process where meaning is constructed by negotiation between the participants. We assume that both participants are actively reflectively and analytically working throughout the interview to determine where the talk should go, and how it should be understood, layer by layer.

Both the traditional empirical approach and the IPA approach use interview as a data collection device, but that is where the similarity ends. Not because one approach is structured and the other allows a structure to emerge, but because the two approaches are underpinned by divergent understandings of the nature of the interview, the nature of the interviewee and the task of knowledge production.

It is relatively easy to appreciate the difference between these two approaches, so we will complicate things by bringing in a third, Inductive Thematic Analysis (ITA, see Chapter 15). Many researchers find it difficult to pick apart the difference between ITA and IPA. Although IPA brings with it different rules about sampling, the focused but open and often brief interview schedule work well with both approaches because both aim to generate lengthy, deep and reflective exploration of participants' experiences. The steps involved in analysing the data (Hayes, 2000; Smith, 1995; Willig, 2001) also look very, very similar (as there are only so many things you can do with interview data). So, where does the difference lie? IPA is interested in the phenomenology of the individual. The analysis begins with the individual and the researcher stays very close to the data of each individual for as long as possible. There is no hurry to look across the data to find pattern, although eventually this is done. ITA is more likely to involve taking the participants words at face value. The interpretation tends to happen at the later stages of analysis rather than at the point of trying to work out what a participant means. Instead, ITA focuses from the outset on moving across the data to find common themes. We have focused on the difference between two approaches here, but the interview would look different again if adopted with the context of a social constructionist or discourse analysis approach (see Chapters 11 and 13).

The crucial difference between the two approaches is not so apparent in the way in which the data are collected, but is visible in the different layers and stages of analysis. Understanding the assumptions behind each approach is crucial when conducting the interview if we are to have data that can be analysed appropriately. If we do not interpret in the interview and follow through appropriately in our questioning we may not be able to understand the individual's meaning well enough to perform the IPA analysis. If we follow each individual's path through the interview too closely and in too much idiosyncratic detail we may not have the kind of data that allows us to look across the group, compare responses and find common ground for our ITA.

Therefore, it does not make sense to talk about methods of data collection separately from research methodologies, as the actions involved in collecting data take on very different meanings from the standpoint of different methodologies and when the epistemological underpinnings of research are examined. The meaning really is within the method (Tseelon, 1991).

Will the Data Collection Method Suit the Participant Group and Their Abilities and Interests?

It is all very well making sure that we as researchers are clear about how our data collection methods answer our research question and connect with our epistemological approach, but we also need to remember that our choice of method also structure the experience our participants. Different data collection methods make different demands on research participants. Researchers need to be aware of these demands and be able to make judgements (preferably in consultation with service users) about whether the methods will place unreasonable or unnecessary burdens on research participants. We also need to consider whether participants have the skills and capabilities necessary to engage with these methods, or whether we need to adapt the method to suit our participants.

Diaries, for example, require literacy skills and certain physical abilities. Where participants lack these skills researchers have to creatively adapt the method to suit participants' needs by collecting audio or video diaries, using webcams or telephones for participants to submit entries, or using online blogs. Participants may need time to 'build rapport' with a data collection technique, becoming familiar with what is expected and what they feel comfortable revealing, just as they need to develop a relationship with the researcher (Jacelon & Imperio, 2005).

Focus groups are often praised as providing an opportunity for participants to share their experiences and difficulties within a potentially supportive environment of others (Frith, 2000; Kreuger, 2008), but finding a time and place to meet everyone's needs can be challenging. This might not suit client groups whose lives are chaotic as they will be unlikely to turn up at the right time or place to take part in the research. It may also not suit clients who are socially anxious or unwilling to share their views in front of other people. However, working flexibly and innovatively with the method can reap rewards. For example, young people who experience chronic skin conditions may find it difficult to articulate their experiences in face-to-face meetings with others, but participating in online group discussions may allow the same elements of support to arise whilst avoiding the difficulties of managing appearance issues (Fox et al., 2007). Email interviews, telephone interviews or written blogs may provide similar strategies for managing this issue.

Similarly, the relatively unstructured interviews often used in IPA for collecting rich narratives about individual experience require participants to be effective and articulate storytellers, willing and able to share their experiences in a narrative form. This may make the method unsuitable for groups of participants who may be less familiar with sharing their views in this way and may provide brief and less articulate responses. This is not to say that this kind of interviewing should never be used with these groups, but it may be appropriate to think creatively about how a relatively open and unstructured interview could be conducted effectively. For example, it might be appropriate to use visual methods such as photographs or drawings to help participants orientate to the topic under discussion, to make abstract concepts more concrete and to enable them to express their views fully. Frith and Harcourt (2007) found that using photo-diaries to capture women's experience of chemotherapy treatment allowed them to produce more elaborated accounts of their illness experience, and to capture their changing experiences over time. Similarly, Johnson (2010) found that using photographs in a participatory action research project with lesbian, gay, bisexual and transgender young people with mental health difficulties not only helped these young people to talk about their experiences, but also provided a vivid and engaging way to communicate the results of the research. If you have the vision to use this method creatively, the skills to be able to facilitate the method effectively and the confidence to justify your approach, then this would be the right one for your research question. Another approach would be to use memories as triggers for eliciting narratives as is the case in memory work (for an example of memory work see Gillies *et al.*, 2004). In all these cases, the aim is to encourage participants to talk about their experiences as openly as possible in a way that is best suited to them and the aims of the research. These accounts can be facilitated with a range of different techniques from the much used interview schedule to the less commonly used photograph or memory.

How Does the Method Structure the Process of Engagement?

Different methods of data collection structure a different relationship and level of engagement between researcher and participant along a dimension from 'experimenter as a stimulus' at one end, through 'collaboration' to 'participant led' at the other pole. Why is this important? It will certainly affect the willingness of participants to engage with our research. Although some participants may not be in a sufficiently powerful position to resist the research efforts of mental health researchers, they may be pretty unforthcoming about their experiences.

Qualitative research almost always involves an interaction between the researcher and the participant, but this is sometimes a close and intense interaction, and sometimes distant. You could be researching yourself as a practitioner, leading research as a service user and drawing on your own experience for data or undergoing the prolonged and intense engagement required by ethnography. Embedded in this might be ideas about attempting to empower participants, to manage power relations or carry out ethical research. But even more typical methods, such as the one-to-one interview, invite the participant and the researcher to work together to generate data. In all of these methods, concerns with power, ethics and politics shape decisions about the relationship between the researcher and the researched.

Using focus groups to explore the stigma associated with schizophrenia, Schulze and Angermeyer (2003) argued that the method created multiple lines of communication between participants who share experiences. As such, the dynamics of the group decreased the influence of the researcher, allowing participants' voices to gain more prominence. Other methods, such as the collection of naturalistically occurring interactions (such as between therapists and patients, family members or members of a support group) or the use of existing documents (policy documents, archives of

Internet discussions), require very little (or even no) engagement between researcher and participant. When McCabe *et al.* (2002) used conversation analysis to explore recordings of appointments in outpatient psychiatric clinics they were able to identify how patients' attempts to initiate conversations about the content of their psychotic symptoms often evoked hesitation from psychiatrists who avoided giving answers even to direct questions. Although this method requires minimal involvement from participants, it may be a way of including those who are typically unlikely to volunteer to take part in interviews, as their involvement requires no additional time or resources. These methods may not seek to 'empower' participants through collaborative research, but may reveal the operation of power in the everyday lives of service users and how mental health interventions occur in practice rather than in theory. Another example of a research method that involves minimal engagement from participants is web-based research that analyses Internet discussion groups in which the 'data' is produced for a purpose other than research (Hewson, 2002; James, 2009). For example, Gavin *et al.* (2008) were able to analyse postings to an online 'pro-anorexia' discussion forum and examine the ways in which members of the forum created a group identity without placing any additional burden on the contributors.

Issues of engagement are not just a byproduct of the method adopted. It is the ethical and political commitments of the researcher that may shape the way in which they approach research design and this may be central to the method that they seek to adopt. Fortunately, there is also an increasing pressure to adopt methods and ways of conducting research and collecting data that incorporates service user involvement (see Chapter 4).

How Will my Participants Make Sense of This Method?

Participants often misunderstand aspects of research process, making issues of informed consent problematic. We need to think carefully not only about how methods of data collection are explained to individuals, but also to try to anticipate how they might make sense of the research tasks in which they are being invited to engage. When meeting novel experiences we draw on what we already know to make sense of a situation and to figure out how to behave.

Research interviews, for example, can mirror therapeutic encounters because both provide space for people to talk about their experiences with someone who wants to listen, and require similar skills of listening and attending to participants' responses (Tee & Lathlean, 2004). Schulze and Angermeyer (2003) argued that the people with a diagnosis of schizophrenia who took part in their study might be intimidated by the interview situation, reminded of therapeutic relationships, and consequently adjust their communication perhaps expecting to receive expert knowledge, help and advice. They opted for focus groups instead, but this might be just as likely to be confused with a group therapy session.

When researchers take time and trouble to build relationships there is a danger that participants may misconstrue the research experience as an opportunity to develop true friendships. Many researchers adopt well-documented strategies to enhance rapport – such as sharing a meal, attending family gatherings, looking at family photos and running errands (Dickson-Swift *et al.*, 2006). These activities, especially when coupled with the in-depth sharing of feelings, attitudes and beliefs characteristic of an interview, are usually a feature of intimate relationships. While rapport may facilitate the telling of stories, researchers also need to balance this against their own objectivity, the possibility that participants may not understand the non-reciprocal nature of the interview and the prospect of researcher burnout. Where rapport is at its strongest, that exploitation of relationships is of greatest concern.

These dilemmas come into sharper focus when using methods that require deeper and more prolonged levels of engagement between the researcher and participants such as ethnography, longitudinal research involving multiple interviews, or biographical research which may follow a small number of individuals very intensely. While therapists and practitioners may be well accustomed to thinking about how to manage boundary issues with clients, they may be less aware of how these issues may play out in relation to research participants (for further discussion of the ethical dilemmas involved in qualitative research see Chapter 3).

It is important to remember that however we seek to position ourselves in research (as confidants, benignly curious or facilitating empowerment), our participants will be actively trying to work out who we are, what we represent and why we want the knowledge that we are asking for. In an ideal world there might be a close fit between how we represent ourselves and how we are seen by participants; however, it is often not a perfect world. Participants may be actively mistrustful of our motivations and interpret our presence as threatening. Receiving vague answers to questions posed to young people about drug use or people with learning difficulties about their sexual behaviour may be an indication that they see the questions as a threat. Providing brief reticent vague answers may be in their interests because knowledge about their sexual and drug-related behaviour may lead to interference from others. A useful question to ask oneself is: How will my participants interpret my role? Why do they think that I want this information and what do they think I will do with it?

Consultation with service users raises a complex set of issues. Apart from establishing whether the aims of the research coincide with their aims, and whether they feel that the research is empowering to them (we often assume that allowing a voice to be heard is inherently empowering, but people with less power do not inevitably gain when they share their knowledge and insight about their own experience with others who are in a position of power) we then have to face the question of whether the method is meaningful to the participants. Are they able and willing to share in the aims of the project in order to provide data that is suited to the analytic method we intend to use and capable of answering our research question?

Conclusions

Deciding which method of data collection to use is only part of the planning and decision making that underpins data collection. Thinking about how to implement this method, and how to present it to research participants is just as important. This leads on to a range of issues which fall outside of the umbrella of data collection techniques, but which do affect the ways in which participants experience and understand those techniques. These include a range of self-presentational issues about dress, participant information sheets, how the researcher introduces themselves, and defines their role and occupational title; and how they conduct the recruitment and consenting procedures. All the time that the researcher is juggling these issues they are also actively trying to pin down their own epistemological, ethical, political and professional positions. Rather than try to resolve all these issues, we will draw attention to them, and to the questions that they raise, in the form of a summary table (Table 5.1).

Table 5.1   Table showing the relationship between specific data collection approaches, compatibility with epistemological positions, limitations and the skills required for use

Data collection approach	Compatible epistemology	Data format	Participant skills	Advantages	Disadvantages
One-to-one interviews	Any from positivist/ traditional empirical approaches to social constructionist	Verbatim transcripts Partial transcripts, audio and video	Ability to communicate in interview with or without interpreter	Each participant's view is included Opportunity to explore an individual's perspective and in their own terms Access to phenomenology of the individual Participant has relatively high degree of control	Can be an intensive and intrusive experience Can be difficult to clarify the status of the relationship between interviewer and interviewee
Focus groups	Any from positivist/ traditional empirical approaches to social constructionist	Verbatim transcripts Partial transcripts, audio and video	Ability to communicate in interview with or without interpreter Ability to contribute in complex social interaction	Can encourage participants who feel reticent about expressing their views to talk Hearing other views can stimulate discussion and allow elaboration and evaluation of contributions	Can be difficult to keep the group on topic Can be difficult to access minority perspectives Can be uncomfortable for participants

Table 5.1   (*Continued*)

Data collection approach	Compatible epistemology	Data format	Participant skills	Advantages	Disadvantages
Email interviews	Any from positivist/ traditional empirical approaches to social constructionist	Written content of emails	Ability to communicate in writing, ability to use computer package and computer	Great focus on the individual participant Participant has scope to review and revise their statements High level of participant control Easy to assess participant's ongoing consent Data is ready transcribed and therefore easily prepared	Can be technically difficult The lengthy process can lead to participant withdrawal It may be difficult to ensure confidentiality It can be difficult to build rapport with participants Time gaps between responses can lead to lack of spontaneity, forgetting of issues that were discussed and loss of rapport
Solicited diaries	Any from positivist/ traditional empirical approaches to social constructionist	Written, verbatim transcripts, audio and video Visual data	Ability to use designated means for recording diary	Great scope for individual expression and creativity in recording material	Difficult to ensure diaries are completed and that the researcher has access to them
Recordings of naturalistic interactions	Any from positivist/ traditional empirical approaches to social constructionist	Verbatim transcripts Partial transcripts, audio and video	Ability to communicate in conversation with or without interpreter	Less concern about researcher intrusion into data	Harder to explore research questions exhaustively as the researcher cannot direct conversations and the nature of material discussed

(*Continued*)

Table 5.1   (*Continued*)

Data collection approach	Compatible epistemology	Data format	Participant skills	Advantages	Disadvantages
Ethnography	Social constructionist and phe-nomenological approaches	Verbatim transcripts Partial transcripts, audio and video, written field notes	Ability to take part in social events being observed, ability to communicate with researcher	Good scope for exploring phenomenology Allows surprise data to emerge	Potentially very lengthy and time-consuming Requires a great deal of skill from the researcher
Internet-based research	Any from positivist/traditional empirical approaches to social constructionist	Written verbatim transcripts of online discussions	Ability to use computers and express oneself in written form	Less concern about researcher intrusion into data No additional burden on participants May access hard-to-reach groups	Harder to explore research questions exhaustively as the researcher cannot direct conversations and the nature of material discussed
Visual methods	Any from positivist/traditional empirical approaches to social constructionist	Photographs, paintings, drawings, etc., usually accompanied by transcripts of written/verbal narratives	Ability to produce visual materials and often to communicate about these materials in written or verbal form	Allows individual creativity of expression	Hard to analyse without ac-companying narrative

References

Dickson-Swift, V., James, E.L., Kippen, S. & Liamputtong, P. (2006). Blurring boundaries in qualitative health research on sensitive topics. *Qualitative Health Research, 16*, 853–871.

Fox, F., Morris, M. & Rumsey, N. (2007). Doing synchronous online focus groups with young people: Methodological reflections. *Qualitative Health Research, 17*, 539–547.

Frith, H. (2000). Focusing on sex: Using focus groups in sex research. *Sexualities, 3*, 275–297.

Frith, H. & Harcourt, D. (2007). Using photographs to capture women's experiences of chemotherapy: Reflecting on the method. *Qualitative Health Research, 17,* 1340–1350.

Gavin, J., Rodham, D. & Poyer, H. (2008). The presentation of pro-anorexia in online group interactions. *Qualitative Health Research, 18,* 325–333.

Gillies, V., Harden, A., Johnson, K., Reavey, P., Strange, V. & Willig, C. (2004). Women's collective constructions of embodied practices through memory work: Cartesian dualism in memories of sweating and pain. *British Journal of Social Psychology, 43,* 99–113.

Hayes, N. (2000). *Thematic qualitative analysis in doing psychological research.* London: Sage.

Hewson, C. (2002). *Internet research methods: A practical guide for social and behavioural researchers.* London: Sage.

Jacelon, C.J. & Imperio, K. (2005). Participant diaries as a source of data in research with older adults. *Qualitative Health Research, 15,* 991–997.

James, N. (2009). *Online interviewing.* London: Sage.

Johnson, K. (2010). Witnessing, wit(h)nessing and social activism: Some theoretical reflections on the transformative possibilities of participatory visual methodologies. Paper presented at the Social Life of Methods Conference, Oxford, UK, August 2010.

Kinsey, A.C., Pomeroy, W. & Martin, C.E. (Eds.) (1948). *Sexual behaviour in the human man.* Philadelphia: WB Saunders.

Kreuger, R.A. (2008). *Focus groups: A practical guide for applied research* (4th edn). London: Sage.

McCabe, R., Heath, C., Burns, T. & Priebe, S. (2002). Engagement of patients with psychosis in the consultation: Conversation analytic study. *British Medical Journal, 325,* 1148–1151.

Schulze, B. & Angermeyer, M.C. (2003). Subjective experiences of stigma: A focus group study of schizophrenic patients, their relatives and mental health professionals. *Social Science and Medicine, 56,* 299–312.

Smith, J.A. (1995). Semi-structured interviewing and qualitative analysis. In J.A. Smith, R. Harre & L. Van Langenhove (Eds.)*Rethinking methods in psychology* (pp. 9–26). London: Sage.

Tee, S.R. & Lathlean, J. (2004). The ethics of conducting a co-operative inquiry with vulnerable people. *Journal of Advanced Nursing, 47,* 536–543.

Tseelon, E. (1991). The method is the message on the meaning of methods as ideologies. *Psychology and Theory, 1,* 299–316.

Willig, C. (2001). Interpretative phenomenological analysis. In *Introducing Qualitative Research in Psychology: Adventures in Theory and Method* (pp. 50–68). Buckingham: Open University Press.

Further reading

Alaszewski, A. (2006). *Using diaries for social research.* London: Sage.

King, N. & Horrocks, C. (2010). *Interviews in qualitative research.* London: Sage.

Madden, R. (2010). Being ethnographic: A guide to the theory and practice of ethnography. London: Sage.

6

Qualitative Methods for Studying Psychotherapy Change Processes

Robert Elliott

Introduction

Originally, research on psychotherapy, counselling and related mental health interventions fell into two divisions: *outcome* research, which dealt with the extent to which clients change over the course of treatment, and *process* research, which investigated what occurs within treatment sessions. *Change process research* (CPR) was proposed by Greenberg (1986) to bridge these two fields, pointing to the need to study the processes that bring about changes, including the temporal course of those changes. Thus, CPR concerns itself with explaining both *how* and *why* change occurs (Elliott, 2010).

It is my hope in this chapter to encourage the use of a broader range of options for qualitative data collection and analysis in CPR. To do this, I first briefly summarize two useful tools for collecting useful and interesting qualitative data about change processes. After this, I turn briefly to an example of qualitative data analysis methods appropriate to CPR. However, prior to doing this I briefly outline some of the epistemological issues associated with CPR.

Epistemological Issues and the History of Change Process Research

In spite of having a great deal of psychological theory about what brings change about, we still know relatively little about how change actually occurs in most mental health interventions, making qualitative discovery-oriented methods especially appropriate.

Qualitative Research Methods in Mental Health and Psychotherapy: A Guide for Students and Practitioners, First Edition.
Edited by D. Harper and A.R. Thompson.
© 2012 John Wiley & Sons, Ltd. Published 2012 by John Wiley & Sons, Ltd.

Traditionally, the mode of understanding assumed to operate in CPR has been realist and causal in nature, as revealed by the use of implicit physicalist metaphors such as 'change mechanisms' (change process as machine) and 'effective ingredients' (a pharmaceutical metaphor).

Accordingly, most CPR to date has been quantitative and hypothesis-testing, reflecting not only the influence of positivism but also researchers' desires to test strong causal theories, such as Rogers' (1957) mechanistic formulation of the necessary and sufficient conditions for change in therapy. Most commonly, researchers have used measures of process such as rating of therapeutic alliance to predict outcome (e.g., questionnaires measuring client distress). For most researchers, causal inference and quantitative assessment have been perceived as tightly linked elements of the standard modus operandi.

In fact, although the process-outcome genre of quantitative CPR has produced large numbers of findings, these have tended toward either restating the obvious (general quality of helping relationship is important) or have resulted in contradictory results (cf. Shapiro *et al.* 1994). Furthermore, Stiles and Shapiro (1989) have strongly criticized the quantitative process-outcome paradigm on various grounds, mostly having to do with the simplistic assumptions it makes about the nature of the therapy process (e.g., if something is good, then more of it must always be better; i.e., the dose–response metaphor). Even at their best, quantitative process-outcome research designs are blunt instruments for understanding anything as complex and nuanced as the process of change in psychotherapy or other mental health interventions. Thus, the vast accumulation of general or contradictory research findings conceals our fundamental ignorance about how individual clients actually grow and change in the course of their therapies. In the absence of careful prior qualitative research, tightly focused process-outcome research is analogous to poking a long stick into a deep hole: if you do it enough times, eventually you will hit something, but you may still not be sure what it is.

In fact, since the mid 1990s, qualitative CPR research studies now appear regularly (e.g., recent special section of *Psychotherapy Research*; see Elliott, 2008). However, Polkinghorne's (1994) lament still holds: the range of qualitative research strategies applied to date has been fairly limited to qualitative interview studies analysed with variations of Grounded Theory or Interpretative Phenomenological Analysis. Thus, the potential of qualitative approaches drawing on hermeneutic, constructivist or social constructionist epistemologies remains to be fully tapped. Specifically, narrative, conversation and discourse analysis approaches to CPR on mental health treatments have so far been under-utilized.

Research Questions in Change Process Research

By definition, qualitative CPR is organized around a central research question: how does change occur in some particular mental health intervention? This then opens up into several subsidiary and partially overlapping research questions, each of which points to a different genre or approach to CPR (whose strengths and limitations have recently been reviewed by Elliott, 2010):

- What factors (i.e., client, therapist or relational processes) bring about client change (*helpful factors* research)?
- Which client processes are facilitated by which therapist responses under which conditions (discourse analytic or micro-analytic *sequential process* research)?
- What happens in important episodes of therapeutic change (*significant events* research)?

Each of these genres of CPR has an emerging body of research around it. Cutting across each of these research genres are sets of still more detailed research questions that follow from a broad orienting framework of the change process in mental health interventions (Elliott, 1991). These include the role of the different *parties* (or persons) to the therapeutic process:

- What *therapist* processes facilitate client change?
- What *client* processes (types of action, content, style/manner or skillfulness) facilitate (or constitute) client change?
- What *relational* processes facilitate client change?
  Furthermore, the framework also identifies research questions corresponding to the main *phases* surrounding the change process:
- What *contexts* (immediate or more distant) precede change processes?
- What are the *effects* (immediate or delayed) of a particular change process?

Any of these research questions can be asked of the different *perspectives* on the therapeutic process: how do *client, therapist* or *research/third party observers* perceive these processes? Finally, we might want to know what a particular change process looks like at different levels of resolution within the intervention we are studying: *speaking turn, episode* (i.e., a coherent sequence of speaking turns within a session), *session* or *relationship* as whole. Clearly, there is great scope for CPR.

Collecting Change Process Research Data

The possibilities for collecting qualitative data on change processes are numerous, including post-treatment interviews (e.g., the Change Interview; Elliott *et al.*, 2001), post-session open-ended questionnaires (e.g., the Helpful Aspects of Therapy Form; Llewelyn *et al.*, 1988), therapist process notes and reports (Todd *et al.*, 1992), various forms of open-ended and semi-structured tape-assisted recall interviews (Elliott, 1986; Rennie, 1990) and audio or video recordings of psychotherapy or counselling sessions, which can be transcribed. Similar to other forms of qualitative research, the number of participants depends on several factors, but principally on the purpose of the research, the complexity of the process being studied and the richness of the data collected. First, research attempting to describe a process generally (as opposed to providing an in-depth understanding of one or more single instances) will require more participants of a more diverse character. Secondly, more complex or diverse phenomena will require more participants and longer interviews to represent them effectively. Third, 'thinner' data protocols, such as post-therapy self-report questionnaires, and rarer phenomena, such as hindering processes, will require substantially more informants. Generally, however, the number of informants involved, and the amount of data collected from each, is a function of how many data it takes before one stops finding new categories (types or aspects) for the phenomenon. This point of diminishing returns is generally referred to as *saturation* (Strauss & Corbin, 1998), although it is important to recognize that this is always a matter of degree.

The Research Alliance in CPR is particularly worthy of mention, as in any form of applied social science research, relevant codes of ethical practice are followed in qualitative CPR, based on the core ethical values of beneficence, non-maleficence, autonomy, fidelity and justice (Kitchener, 1984). More specifically, following Mearns and McLeod (1984), the principles of Person-Centred Therapy apply equally to in qualitative CPR, especially those that involve direct interaction with participants (as opposed to discourse or text-based methods):

1. *Empathy*. The researcher focuses on understanding, from the inside, the research participant's lived experiencing.
2. *Unconditional Positive Regard*. The researcher accepts, does not judge and even prizes the research participant's experiencing.
3. *Genuineness*. The researcher tries to be an authentic and equal partner with the research participant, treating them as a co-researcher and allowing them to see the researcher as a fellow human being.
4. *Flexibility*. The researcher creatively and flexibly adapts research methods to the research topic and questions at hand.

These principles form the basis of the Research Alliance in CPR, comparable in some ways to the therapeutic alliance in mental health interventions, although there are some important differences (for further discussion of the ethical issues associated with the research relationship see Chapter 3). At the same time, CPR offers a natural strategy for systematically involving mental health service users in the evaluation of their care, providing them with a voice that both allows them to speak in their own words and that can be validated by the use of systematic, scientifically rigorous procedures. In fact, I would argue that the Helpful Aspects of Therapy Form and the Change Interview, both described below, should be used more often as vehicles for enabling mental health service users to have their voice heard. This could be done by offering them to service user organizations and advocacy groups.

Examples of Qualitative Change Process Research Data Collection Methods

I begin with examples of two qualitative data collection methods that lend themselves to therapy CPR: the Helpful Aspects of Therapy (HAT) Form, a post-session self-report measure, and the Change Interview, an open-ended interview.

Helpful Aspects of Therapy Form

The significant events approach to CPR (Rice & Greenberg, 1984; Stiles *et al.*, 1986) arose as an approach to understanding the immediate effects (*micro-outcomes*) of important moments in psychotherapy or counselling. As such, it contrasts with research that addresses the overall change process in therapy, as assessed by the Change Interview (see next section). Features of significant events research include: (i) focus on clinically significant change events; (ii) simplification by limiting investigation to relatively homogeneous classes of events (e.g. insight events); and (iii) description of the therapeutic sequences by which clients accomplish specific therapeutic tasks within sessions (e.g., exploring and symbolizing trauma-related fears). Although therapist versions of the HAT exist, client-identified significant events are a crucial component of the Events Paradigm, exemplified by the two qualitative data collection methods discussed here.

The HAT Form (Llewelyn *et al.*, 1988) is a mostly qualitative post-session self-report questionnaire which uses open-ended questions to help clients write down their experiences of helpful and hindering therapy events. It is the most frequently employed method for identifying and collecting significant events for further analysis. The HAT is a simple and efficient means of soliciting information from clients about their perceptions of key change processes in therapy. Solicited accounts methods such as the HAT Form are more feasible, less intrusive and create less reactivity than more exhaustive methods such as the tape-assisted recall (Elliott, 1986). The HAT's open-ended format generates qualitative data of sufficient detail and focus that it lends itself to various uses, including identification of significant events, descriptive and interpretive forms of qualitative data analysis and even quantitative content analysis (e.g., Castonguay *et al.*, 2010).

The HAT Form is typically completed by clients either immediately following therapy sessions or within a day of the session, in order to be able to recall it clearly. Most clients complete it without much difficulty, although it does require more time (roughly 5–10 minutes) and effort than quantitative rating scales. It is common for it to be administered following every session, providing a naturalistic account of client perceptions of significant events over the course of therapy. Under these conditions, filling out the HAT Form becomes a routine part of the client's overall therapy experience, and appears to help clients process their therapy more effectively. The most common problems appear to be responses that are very brief, vague or global. Another issue is that client and therapist descriptions of significant events often do not agree (e.g., Caskey *et al.*, 1984)

The descriptive data generated by the HAT Form appear to fall into several general types of information, including within-session *processes*; immediate client *reactions*;

and, less commonly, *contextual* information. For example, after her fifth session, a client whom I will call Rachel wrote the following on her HAT Form:

> *Helpful event:* I placed the center of my fears in my gut [= process]. They were more abstract and therefore more uncontrollable before [= context].
>
> *Why it was helpful:* It gave me a definite 'thing' to overcome [= reaction] rather than external, all encompassing overwhelming fear [= context].
>
> *Helpfulness rating:* 8.5 (between greatly and extremely helpful)
>
> *Where in session:* (blank)
>
> *Length of event:* (blank)
>
> *Other helpful events:* no
>
> *Hindering events:* no

The example given illustrates the usefulness of HAT event descriptions. First, the description was specific enough for a researcher to use it to identify the significant event on the session recording. Secondly, it is detailed enough to enable readers to understand the kind of therapeutic event referred to even without access to the session recording. Thirdly, it also provides information about the client's internal experience that might not have been so easy to infer from the recording. Fourthly, it offers a mini-narrative of a change process that reveals the sequence of client change. Finally, scanning such HAT protocols after therapy is over can enable a therapist very quickly to gain an overview of their client's view of the highpoints of their therapy.

The Change Interview

As can be seen in Table 6.1, the Change Interview (Elliott *et al.*, 2001) assesses several kinds of information; its central purpose, however, is to obtain clients' understandings of what has changed and how those changes have come about, including factors that have interfered with change. The Change Interview first provides a qualitative evaluation of outcome, to complement the widespread predominance of quantitative outcome assessment (McLeod, 2000), offering access to changes that may be missed by traditional measures. The interview offers a chance for clients to explain these changes in their own words and in so doing allows them an opportunity to reflect on and find words for these changes. The process therefore not only provides researchers with valuable information, but also helps clients to assimilate therapeutic work.

The Change Interview attempts to work against the researcher's likely expectations that psychotherapy or counselling will be helpful and that client change is primarily brought about by formal mental health intervention (cf. Elliott, 2002). Thus, it probes in multiple ways for negative changes or hindering or missing factors, as well as positive changes or helpful factors. Similarly, the interview deliberately seeks information about non-therapy factors in client change. Beyond adding credibility, these kinds of information are valuable for improving therapy and locating it in a broader context

Table 6.1 Change interview outline (2008 version, abbreviated)

1. *General experience of therapy.* What has therapy been like for you (so far)?
2. *Changes.* What *changes*, if any, have you noticed in yourself since therapy started?
3. *Change ratings. Expectedness, likelihood without therapy,* and *importance* of each change (5-point rating scales).
4. *Attributions.* In general, what do you *attribute* these various changes to?
5. *Resources.* What *personal strengths* or aspects of your current *life situation* have helped you make use of therapy to deal with your problems?
6. *Limitations.* What things about *you* or your *life situation* have made it harder for you to use therapy to deal with your problems?
7. *Helpful aspects.* What have been the most *helpful* things about your therapy so far?
8. *Problematic aspects.* What kinds of things about the therapy have been *hindering,* unhelpful, negative or disappointing for you? Was there anything that was *difficult* or *missing* from your treatment?
9. *Research aspects.* What has it been like for you to be involved in this research?

© R. Elliott (2008)

(cf. Dreier, 2008). These aspects of the Change Interview reflect its use as an essential component of Hermeneutic Single Case Efficacy Design (HSCED), a complex, mixed method approach to evaluating causality in single treatment cases (Elliott, 2002).

The Change Interview is partially structured by the interview guide in Table 6.1, but researchers are encouraged to adopt an attitude of curiosity, using both open-ended exploratory questions and empathic understanding responses to help the client elaborate their experiences. In general, the client is asked to provide as much detail as possible. The Change Interview is best administered at the end of therapy and at regular intervals throughout treatment (e.g., every 10 sessions). Although it is often a demanding experience for clients, it provides an invaluable opportunity to understand change from the client's point of view.

The following example is an excerpt from a Change Interview administered after session 8. The client, whom we referred to as Rachel in the previous section, was an 18-year-old woman with crime-related post-traumatic stress disorder (PTSD), seen in Emotion-focused therapy. The focus of therapy was her pervasive and extremely debilitating fear. Here are some excerpts from her interview, in which she refers to the same significant event identified by HAT Form after session 5:

> Rachel: I could never comprehend that you could stop fear because, I couldn't control it. When I was afraid, I was afraid, and it's like really helped me, it's like he's almost *making me identify it [the fear] as a solid object inside of me, something that can be rid.* And *it helps to know that in the future, maybe it is something I could overcome.* I never thought that my fear would be something I could overcome . . . [Another change is] *it makes me think more rational thoughts.* . . . And even though I could tell myself, 'That's not reality, there's no one in this house', . . . it's like I could never believe the rational part of me. And it's almost like *doing all this has almost made me rationalize, like 'No, there's no one here', and believe it a little better, and calm down a little more.* So yeah, I noticed differences.

Rachel's responses add to our understanding of her experience of the change process. She describes specific examples of two changes resulting from the therapy process, noted in italics above. In addition, this example provides feedback about a helpful aspect of therapy.

Qualitative Data Analysis Options

Medium-sized sets of data generated from multiple cases using the HAT Form, the Change Interview and other CPR data collection methods such as tape-assisted recall can be analysed using any of the standard systematic qualitative data analysis methods common today, such as Grounded Theory Analysis (especially the Rennie *et al.*, 1988, adaptation; see also Chapter 10) or Interpretative Phenomenological Analysis (Smith *et al.*, 2009; see also Chapter 8). Similarly, smaller data sets of meaning-rich data such as HAT descriptions or transcripts of significant events can be usefully analysed with Discourse Analysis (e.g., Madill & Barkham, 1997) or Conversation Analysis (e.g., Viklund *et al.*, 2010). Many or most of these will be familiar to readers from other chapters in this book and elsewhere. Therefore, I will focus on a less-known form of analysis appropriate for transcripts of significant events: Task Analysis (Rice & Greenberg, 1984; Greenberg, 2007).

Task analysis of significant events

Task analysis is a rational-empirical approach developed by cognitive psychologists for studying how people carry out problem-solving tasks (Ericsson & Simon, 1984). Rice and Greenberg (1984; Greenberg, 2007) adapted the method for studying how clients successfully resolve emotional processing difficulties in therapy. As originally proposed by Rice and Greenberg (1984), task analysis emphasized the later stage of quantitative analysis. Here, in contrast, I emphasize the initial qualitative analysis, which involves careful but open clinical qualitative analysis of interaction sequences in significant events.

Therapeutic Task Analysis assumes that significant events have the following general formal structure, comparable to axial coding domains in Grounded Theory:

- A *marker*, signalling the client's experiential state of readiness to work on a thera-peutic task, that is, a particular unresolved problem or issue (e.g., an internal conflict between contradictory wishes).
- A client *performance model* of the steps through which the client moves toward resolution (e.g., enactment of internal dialogue between conflicting wishes).
- *Therapist responses* that facilitate client performance (e.g., Gestalt two chair work).
- A *task resolution*, in the form of meaningful therapeutic change (e.g., integration of conflicting wishes).

Returning again to the client Rachel's significant event from session 5, Elliott *et al.* (2001) carried out a qualitative Task Analysis by first articulating a rudimentary *rational model* of the marker, client steps, end state and therapist facilitating actions for empathic exploration, based on an earlier formulation of the 'empathic exploration' task (which space precludes presenting). The second step in a task analysis is to collect examples of successful resolutions. For this example, Elliott *et al.* (2001) used the transcript of a significant event in which Rachel identified her 'fear-thing' as the source of her PTSD. The third step was to develop an intensive qualitative description of the sequence from marker to resolution. In this case, the researchers put their preliminary rational model 'in brackets' and attempted to develop an individualized understanding of the process involved in this significant event. Thus, they conducted a qualitative, turn-by-turn analysis of the sequence of client and therapist responses in the event. To do this, each of the three authors separately characterized the series of relevant client and therapist responses, then met to develop a consensus version of the sequence.

Finally, the results of the qualitative sequence analysis were used to modify the initial rational model, yielding a much more detailed revised task model, as presented in Table 6.2 including revised, more precise client marker (referred to as presentation of *undifferentiated client experience*) and performance model, featuring three phases (*task initiation, exploration work* and *closure work*). In addition, the researchers examined the therapist's responses in order to generate a set of specific therapist treatment principles, which became the revised therapist responses part of the model. Finally, they revised the description of client resolution, in the form of a *clarification of a key client emotion scheme*.

The revised task model presented here needs further study with additional significant events, the usual procedure in Task Analysis, cycling between evolving model and concrete examples, until the model appears reasonably stable.

Discussion: Issues in Qualitative Change Process Research

Quality criteria for qualitative Change Process Research

What makes for good qualitative CPR? Of course, this depends on the standards of good practice specific to the particular qualitative research genre and the data collection and analysis procedures employed. For the most part, these standards are the same as those proposed by Elliott *et al.* (1999; e.g., ground themes/categories in examples; promote experiential validity; see also Chapter 16).

Ultimately, qualitative CPR must be judged against the ambitions of CPR in general; helping us to understand how particular kinds of change occur in psychotherapy and other mental health interventions. Thus, the results of CPR studies must go beyond the broad scientific goals of definition and description in order to provide guiding explanations and practical applications. In other words, does this study give us a better understanding of how it works?; does it help us do a better job with our clients? For example, the Task Analysis of Rachel's empathic exploration of her trauma-related fear

Table 6.2   Revised Task Analytic model of empathic exploration for undifferentiated experiences

---

A.   *Marker: Exploration object/issue* (e.g., 'It' marker), which is:
   1.   Undifferentiated (e.g., abstract, unclear)
   2.   Disowned or distanced (e.g., 'It', 'thing')
   3.   Indicated by client to have personal significance (e.g., relevance to presenting problem, identity)
B.   *Client Performance Process*:
   1.   *Task initiation.* C & T identify a particular C experience as a mental 'object'
   2.   *Exploration work* includes at least some of the following sets of meanings (in varying degrees of completeness):
      (a)   Descriptive nature of experience (emotions, bodily sensations, qualities)
      (b)   Relations to other experiences (sources/origins, situational context, effects/functions)
      (c)   Higher order meanings (significance, identity)
      (d)   (Toward end of exploration) Client action-related meanings (wishes, needs, action tendencies)
   3.   *Closure work*: C, T review importance and main points of object definition
C.   *Therapist operations*: Explore multiple aspects of exploration object/issue (not necessarily in sequence):
   •   attune to C internal frame of reference
   •   communicate understanding of C experience
   •   direct C attention to range of aspects of experience (e.g., emotions, bodily experiences, sources, action tendencies)
   •   heighten C experience with repetition and imagery
   •   help C describe emotional experience (e.g., with metaphors, empathic conjectures)
D.   *End state* (resolution): C provides some indication that the experience has shifted
   1.   C feels experience is better defined or specified
   2.   C develops increased reflective distance, disembedding from issue/object
   3.   May include the following as well:
      •   issue/object may be perceived as less threatening or disconcerting for C; C has sense of potential mastery, empowerment
      •   experience may be owned or internalized by client
      •   C may indicate readiness to move on, make changes
      •   C may report feeling better, clearer

Abbreviated from Elliott, R., Slatick, E., & Urman, M. (2001). Qualitative change process research on psychotherapy: Alternative strategies. In J. Frommer and D.L. Rennie (Eds.), *Qualitative psychotherapy research: Methods and methodology* (pp. 69–111). Lengerich, Germany: Pabst Science Publishers.

was the basis for a revised model of that process in Elliott *et al.*'s (2003) emotion-focused therapy manual.

CPR and evidence-based practice

I have recently argued that randomized clinical trials do not constitute a sufficient basis for evidence-based practice, because they focus narrowly on establishing the *existence* of a causal relationship between a mental health intervention and client change, but do not specify the *nature* of that relationship (Elliott, 2010). Mental health interventions are complex conglomerations of intertwined relational and technical elements. Knowing that a type of therapy is associated causally with positive client outcome does not tell us what specifically in that therapy clients use to bring about change in themselves. For this, we need the various forms of CPR: quantitative process-outcome studies, qualitative helpful factors research, micro-analytic discourse analysis of therapeutic sequences and comprehensive analyses of significant change events (e.g., Task Analysis). In fact, truly evidence-based practice should be based on multiple lines of CPR evidence.

Whither qualitative Change Process Research?

In spite of their inherent potential to support clinical practice, CPR methods are: (i) under-utilized; (ii) too often restricted to one particular research design; and (iii) need to be used in concert (Elliott, 2010). It appears to me that the range of qualitative CPR methods currently being employed in the published literature is gradually broadening beyond Grounded Theory analysis, and so on, of qualitative interview data to include, for example, Conversation Analysis (e.g., Viklund *et al.*, 2010), Comprehensive Process Analysis (Elliott *et al.*, 1994) and HSCED (Elliott, 2002), among others. Generic CPR research such as Rennie's (1990) classic study of client in-session experience has been carried out, and we are now seeing the emergence of research on the experiences of particular kinds of clients or particular kinds of therapy (Elliott, 2008). A related current development is the emergence of qualitative meta-synthesis of CPR research, as exemplified by Timulak's (2007) systematic analysis of significant event studies. These methods will enable us to construct generalizable knowledge from disparate studies, even case studies.

What is the future likely to bring? In my view, mainly more and better of the same. However, beyond that, I see continued erosion of the divide between qualitative and quantitative CPR: qualitative themes can be converted into quantitative content analysis categories or rating scales. In addition, quantitative data can be used as pointers toward interesting qualitative phenomena and looked at using a range of qualitative approaches, including both phenomenological-descriptive and social constructionist. CPR researchers will need to learn to be comfortable commuting between qualitative and quantitative methods, even in the same study. Understanding how our clients use their therapy to change themselves requires us to use all available tools.

References

Caskey, N., Barker, C., & Elliott, R. (1984). Dual perspectives: Clients' and therapists' perceptions of therapist responses. *British Journal of Clinical Psychology, 23,* 281–290.

Castonguay, L.G., Boswell, J.F., Zack, S., Baker, S., Boutselis, M., Chiswick, N., *et al.* (2010). Helpful and hindering events in psychotherapy: A practice research network study. *Psychotherapy: Research, Theory, Practice, and Training, 47,* 327–344.

Dreier, O. (2008) *Psychotherapy in everyday life*. Cambridge: Cambridge University Press.

Elliott, R. (1986). Interpersonal Process Recall (IPR) as a psychotherapy process research method. In L. Greenberg & W. Pinsof (Eds.)*The psychotherapeutic process* (pp. 503–527). New York: Guilford.

Elliott, R. (1991). Five dimensions of therapy process. *Psychotherapy Research*, *1*, 92–103.

Elliott, R. (2002). Hermeneutic single case efficacy design. *Psychotherapy Research*, *12*, 1–20.

Elliott, R. (2008). Research on client experiences of therapy: Introduction to the special section. *Psychotherapy Research*, *18*, 239–242.

Elliott, R. (2010). Psychotherapy change process research: Realizing the promise. *Psychotherapy Research*, *20*, 123–135.

Elliott, R., Fischer, C. & Rennie, D. (1999). Evolving guidelines for publication of qualitative research studies in psychology and related fields. *British Journal of Clinical Psychology*, *38*, 215–229.

Elliott, R., Shapiro, D.A., Firth-Cozens, J., Stiles, W.B., Hardy, G., Llewelyn, S.P., *et al.* (1994). Comprehensive process analysis of insight events in cognitive-behavioral and psychodynamic-interpersonal therapies. *Journal of Counseling Psychology*, *41*, 449–463.

Elliott, R., Slatick, E. & Urman, M. (2001). Qualitative change process research on psychotherapy: Alternative strategies. In J. Frommer and D.L. Rennie (Eds.)*Qualitative psychotherapy research: Methods and methodology* (pp. 69–111). Lengerich, Germany: Pabst Science.

Elliott, R., Watson, J.C., Goldman, R.N. & Greenberg, L.S. (2003). *Learning emotion-focused therapy: The process-experiential approach to change*. Washington, DC: APA.

Ericsson, K.A. & Simon, H.A. (1984). *Protocol analysis: Verbal reports as data*. Cambridge: MIT Press.

Greenberg, L.S. (1986). Change process research. *Journal of Consulting and Clinical Psychology*, *54*, 4–9.

Greenberg, L.S. (2007). A guide to conducting a task analysis of psychotherapeutic change. *Psychotherapy Research*, *17*, 15–30.

Kitchener, K.S. (1984). Intuition, critical evaluation and ethical principles: The foundation for ethical decisions in counseling psychology. *Counseling Psychologist*, *12*, 43–55.

Llewelyn, S.P., Elliott, R., Shapiro, D.A., Firth, J. & Hardy, G. (1988). Client perceptions of significant events in prescriptive and exploratory periods of individual therapy. *British Journal of Clinical Psychology*, *27*, 105–114.

Madill, A. & Barkham, M. (1997). Discourse analysis of a theme in one successful case of brief psychodynamic-interpersonal psychotherapy. *Journal of Counseling Psychology*, *44*, 232–244.

McLeod, J. (2000). The contribution of qualitative research to evidence-based counselling and psychotherapy. In N. Rowland & S. Goss (Eds.)*Evidence-based counselling and psychological therapies* (pp. 111–126). London: Routledge.

Mearns, D. & McLeod, J. (1984). A person-centred approach to research. In R.F. Levant & J.M. Shlein (Eds.)*Client centred therapy and the person-centred approach: New directions in theory, research and practice* (pp. 370–389). Eastbourne: Praeger.

Polkinghorne, D.E. (1994). Reaction to special section on qualitative research in counseling process and outcome. *Journal of Counseling Psychology*, *41*, 510–512.

Rennie, D.L. (1990). Toward a representation of the client's experience of the psychotherapy hour. In G. Lietaer, J. Rombauts & R. Van Balen (Eds.)*Client-centered and experiential psychotherapy towards the nineties* (pp. 155–172). Leuven, Belgium: Leuven University Press.

Rennie, D.L., Phillips, J.R. & Quartaro, G.K. (1988). Grounded theory: A promising approach to conceptualization in psychology? *Canadian Psychology, 29,* 139–150.

Rice, L.N. & Greenberg, L. (Eds.) (1984). *Patterns of change.* New York: Guilford Press.

Rogers, C.R. (1957). The necessary and sufficient conditions of therapeutic personality change. *Journal of Consulting Psychology, 21,* 95–103.

Shapiro, D.A., Harper, H., Startup, M., Reynolds, S., Bird, D. & Suokas, A. (1994). The high-water mark of the drug metaphor: A meta-analytic critique of process-outcome research. In R.L Russell (Ed.) *Reassessing psychotherapy research* (pp. 1–35). New York: Guilford.

Smith, J.A., Flowers, P. & Larkin, M. (2009). *Interpretative phenomenological analysis: Theory, method and research.* London: Sage.

Stiles, W.B. & Shapiro, D.A. (1989). Abuse of the drug metaphor in psychotherapy process-outcome research. *Clinical Psychology Review, 9,* 521–543.

Stiles, W.B., Shapiro, D.A. & Elliott, R. (1986). Are all psychotherapies equivalent? *American Psychologist, 41,* 165–180.

Strauss, A. & Corbin, J. (1998). *Basics of qualitative research: Techniques and procedures for developing grounded theory* (2nd edn). Thousand Oaks, CA: Sage.

Timulak, L. (2007). Identifying core categories of client-identified impact of helpful events in psychotherapy: A qualitative meta-analysis. *Psychotherapy Research, 17,* 305–314.

Todd, D.M., Jacobus, S.I. & Boland, J. (1992). Uses of a computer database to support research-practice integration in a training clinic. *Professional Psychology: Research and Practice, 23,* 52–58.

Viklund, E., Holmqvist, R. & Nelson, K.Z. (2010). Client-identified important events in psychotherapy: Interactional structures and practices. *Psychotherapy Research, 20,* 151–164.

Further reading

Elliott, R. (2010). Psychotherapy change process research: Realizing the promise. *Psychotherapy Research, 20,* 123–135.

Elliott, R., Slatick, E. & Urman, M. (2001). Qualitative change process research on psychotherapy: Alternative strategies. In J. Frommer & D.L. Rennie (Eds.) *Qualitative psychotherapy research: Methods and methodology* (pp. 69–111). Lengerich, Germany: Pabst Science.

Greenberg, L.S. (2007). A guide to conducting a task analysis of psychotherapeutic change. *Psychotherapy Research, 17,* 15–30.

7

Choosing a Qualitative Research Method

David Harper

Introduction

For those new to research methods, choosing the most appropriate method of qualitative analysis is often one of the most difficult parts of a research project: there seem to be so many from which to choose and the differences between them can seem opaque. How should one go about the process of choosing? Unfortunately, it is a topic that is often glossed over in many books yet it is often a central concern for academic examiners or journal reviewers. In this chapter I outline some of the things that researchers need to take into account in making a choice.

An important point to make at the start is that this chapter focuses only on choosing a method of data analysis and not of data collection, which was addressed in Chapter 5. Readers might find it helpful to read these chapters in conjunction because, as noted in that chapter, it is important that you collect data that map onto your research questions; sufficiently warrant the kind of claims you wish to make; and match the epistemological assumptions of your method of analysis.

In this chapter, I outline some of the key considerations in choosing a research method and show how different methods are useful for addressing different kinds of research questions.

A Pragmatic Approach to Choosing an Analytic Method

The received view about choosing a method is that it should fit the research question, but that is not the whole story. The proposal here is that choosing a research method is

Qualitative Research Methods in Mental Health and Psychotherapy: A Guide for Students and Practitioners, First Edition.
Edited by D. Harper and A.R. Thompson.
© 2012 John Wiley & Sons, Ltd. Published 2012 by John Wiley & Sons, Ltd.

very much a pragmatic matter and, whilst the research question is important, there are other factors that may need to be considered. For some, the key issue is to clarify one's epistemological assumptions and then choose a research method that is consistent with it. However, this presupposes that one's epistemological stance is not also a matter of choice.

For example, for those training to be therapists or mental health professionals, the primary goal may be educational rather than investigatory – for example, to learn how to use a particular research technique. Priebe and Slade (2006) note that other considerations in choosing an appropriate method might include: the scientific interests of the researcher; their preferences for a particular method; the researcher's expertise in a method; the current popularity of that method; and the relevance of the method to the target audience. Slade and Priebe (2006) note the importance of funding considerations – who will fund the study and in what outcomes are they interested? The audience of an empirical scientific journal will have slightly different expectations from those of an academic examiner. A policy maker, on the other hand, may be more interested in the implications and outcomes of a study and whether it can be generalized to other populations. Service users might be concerned to hear about the involvement of service users in the study (see Chapter 4), that their experience has been understood and that the study will lead to practical changes in services.

Once one has weighed up these considerations one can begin to formulate a research question.

Developing a Research Question

What questions are most suitable for qualitative research? Qualitative methods are, in general, better at developing rich descriptions of phenomena and processes – aiding conceptual and definitional clarification. Common forms of questions include:

- How does the social process occur?
- What are the key elements in experiences of the phenomenon?

Of course, for some researchers, the primary aim may not be to describe an empirical phenomenon, it may be to ask a question underpinned by certain theoretical preoccupations (e.g., feminism, subjectivity, power) and/or drawing on particular theorists (e.g., Foucault, Deleuze, etc.). Thus, one's theoretical and, to some extent, political orientation is also a choice that needs to be made.

As I have noted, each qualitative method has a different focus and, in Box 7.1, we can see the key foci of a range of methods. Readers can look for the focus that seems to encompass their research idea and they can then look in the relevant method chapter and read the section on research questions. Once a method seems appropriate it is advisable to read a number of different empirical examples of the use of that method in order to see the full range of questions that can be addressed.

Be wary of overly broad and vague questions because the danger here is that the decisions about what the analyst is going to focus on are not made explicit and are

Box 7.1 Mapping the Varied Foci of Qualitative Methods

What kind of focus do you wish your study to have?

- Do you want to map out the concourse/terrain/range of ideas/concepts?
  - Q methodology
  - Thematic analysis
- Do you want to summarize unstructured data in thematic categories?
  - Thematic analysis
- Do you want to summarize unstructured data in thematic categories and then represent them numerically or make numerical or quantitative claims (e.g., about the proportions of participants in various categories)?
  - Content analysis
- Do you want to delineate positions participants take up in discourse with a focus on their ideological context/historical emergence?
  - Foucauldian approaches to Discourse Analysis
- Are you interested in the interactional context of talk?
  - Ethnomethodology/Conversation analysis
  - Discursive Psychology approaches to Discourse Analysis
- Do you want to develop a model of social processes?
  - Grounded Theory
- Are you more interested in the subjective experience of the individual?
  - Individual case studies
  - Phenomenology (Interpretative Phenomenological Analysis or Existentialist-informed Phenomenology)
- Are you more interested in the stories individuals and communities tell?
  - Narrative

simply put off until after data collection. A clinical qualitative research question needs to be broad and open-ended but of sufficient clarity and specificity.

Once one has formulated a research question, one then needs to make a final selection of the method, choosing the one that best addresses the question. However, the methods vary in their assumptions and so it is to this issue that we turn next.

Qualitative Methods and Their Assumptions

Many readers more familiar with quantitative research methods will know that there are a variety of different methods that are used to answer particular kinds of question (e.g., covariation, change over time, etc.). Methods only 'work' if certain conditions are met. Qualitative methods differ for exactly the same reasons. First, each is useful in asking different kinds of research question – some focus on individual subjective experience, others investigate social processes, others still examine the societal realm. Secondly, as we saw in Chapter 5, using one kind of method one might assume that what a participant says is a relatively transparent window onto their thoughts and feelings but using a different method one might assume that what people say is much more influenced by the context of the interaction.

In this chapter, I focus on the philosophical assumptions of each method described as a way of differentiating them. A misapprehension which has developed over the years is that there is a major philosophical difference between quantitative and qualitative methods but few between different qualitative methods. However, this is an over-simplification. For instance, as we will see later, not all qualitative methods focus on subjective experience and some would even be sceptical about the concepts used in describing it. Also, in terms of their underlying philosophical assumptions, some qualitative methods have more in common with some quantitative methods than with other qualitative methods.

In a research interview, if a participant says 'I'm happy' and we report that 'the participant is happy' we are making a whole set of assumptions: that the participant has clear knowledge of their emotional state; that they are honestly communicating it to the researcher and so on. However, these assumptions are contestable: participants may think they are happy but the expression on their faces or other indications might suggest otherwise. Similarly, interviewees may be saying they are happy for a variety of reasons in addition to actually being happy: they may not want to burden the interviewer; they may want to close off an area of questioning because they do not feel safe with or do not trust the interviewer; or they may be responding to demand characteristics (Orne, 1962) – implicit role expectations as a result of being participants in a research project.

Just because you want to make a certain claim does not mean it is immune from criticism. Thus, researchers making the assumption that there is a direct correspondence between what participants say and how they subjectively feel need to be able to justify this on the basis of argument and evidence. Similarly, researchers making the assumption that there is no direct correspondence between what is said and experienced need to be able to justify that position. The kind of assumptions researchers make about the relationship between their data and the world are called epistemological assumptions. In Part II there are eight chapters on a range of qualitative methods. In each of these chapters, contributors have helpfully identified the key epistemological assumptions made by that method and so the aim in the next section is to introduce these concepts. For each method it is important to see what research questions it can address and what assumptions it makes. These help us to see what one can (and cannot) claim on the basis of our study when it is written up.

What is Epistemology and Why Does it Matter?

Epistemology is the philosophy of knowledge or 'the study of the nature of knowledge and the methods of obtaining it' (Burr, 2003, p. 202). In other words, it is concerned with research-oriented questions like 'How can I go about gathering knowledge about the world?' and 'How do I know what I know?' Within philosophical debates about knowledge, epistemology is contrasted with ontology which is the 'study of being and existence. The attempt to discover the fundamental categories of what exists' (Burr, 2003, p. 203). The difference can be summarized briefly: epistemology concerns what it is possible to know whereas ontology concerns what there is to know in the world 'out there'.

Different philosophical traditions have answered these questions in different ways. There are different ways of mapping these assumptions and, as Madill and Gough (2008) point out, there are almost as many typologies of qualitative methods as there are authors. For example, Guba and Lincoln (1994) delineate positivism, post-positivism, critical theory and constructivism and examine each with regards to ontology, epistemology and methodology. However, for the sake of simplicity I will, following Willig (in press), focus on three main epistemological frameworks which could be argued to underlie Guba and Lincoln's categorization: realism, phenomenology and social constructionism. There are a number of dimensions that differentiate between these traditions as we will see; however, a key one is the extent to which qualitative data are seen as mirroring and reflecting reality. This is often termed the realism–relativism continuum. Realism is the position that the data collected mirror reality. Relativism, on the other hand, is the position that there are many valid interpretations of the same observation and so data are not seen as directly mirroring reality.

Within each of these traditions, there are variants and I will describe these too as they map more closely onto individual methods in the following sections. Rather more space will be given to social constructionism as there have been vigorous and, to the novice, somewhat confusing debates within this tradition. Although many methods can be differentiated by their underlying epistemological assumptions, some methods can be used from different epistemological standpoints (see Box 7.2).

Box 7.2 The 'Same' Method may be Used by Researchers from Different Epistemological Standpoints

Although it is possible to differentiate methods from each other by their epistemological assumptions, in the case of some methods it is also possible to use the method but from different epistemological standpoints. Thus, Grounded Theory can be used to ask different questions depending on the epistemological framework within which it is used – Madill et al. (2000) analysed interview data from a study where participants were relatives of people with a diagnosis of schizophrenia. The researchers conducted the analysis from three different epistemological positions: realism, contextual constructionism and radical constructionism. As a result, it is important to state one's epistemological assumptions (i.e., which form of a particular method you are using) – for example, whether one is using a realist or social constructionist variant of Grounded Theory (see Chapter 10).

Epistemology underpins knowledge claims not only in research, but also in psychotherapy. As many readers will be familiar with the psychotherapies, I will give examples of psychotherapies that are associated with epistemological frameworks as well as examples of methods. In the section that follows, I will draw heavily on Willig (in press) which is a very clear exposition of debates about epistemology in qualitative research. She also notes how debates about epistemology map onto ethical and political debates in psychology and thus, in trying to identify where you stand epistemologically, you may also need to reflect on your ontological, ethical and political commitments (see also Parker, 2005).

Realism

Researchers working within the realist tradition assume that there is a direct relationship between what is observed and the nature of reality and they assume that the world is rule-bound. As Willig (in press) notes, the aim is 'to generate valid and reliable knowledge about a social and/or psychological phenomenon which exists independently of the researcher's awareness of it'. She argues that the researcher is essentially cast as a detective, attempting to uncover the rules governing social and psychological mechanisms or processes – thus, ethnography and the earlier more realist versions of grounded theory would be located here. For example, Light's (1980) ethnography of the training of US psychiatrists identifies the implicit rules that govern situations like ward rounds, evidencing these claims by citing fieldwork observations and interviews with key participants. Similarly, in ethnomethodology and conversation analysis, there is an attempt to delineate the 'rules' of local interactions.

The vast majority of quantitative research is realist, although few researchers make this assumption explicit because it is taken for granted within mainstream mental health research. There are two subsidiary approaches within the broad realist tradition: direct realism and critical realism.

Direct realism   Direct realists (sometimes called scientific realists or, somewhat pejoratively, 'naive realists') assume that data directly mirror reality. They are thus both ontologically and epistemologically realist. They have, in the past, been referred to as positivists though this is a much misunderstood term (Miller, 1999; Shadish, 1995) and probably best avoided. Shadish (1995) argues that few researchers could be categorized in this way. Some, but not all, behaviour therapists might identify as direct realists.

Critical realism   Critical realists (also termed post-positivists; Guba & Lincoln, 1994) are ontological realists in that they assume that our data can tell us about reality but they do not view this as a direct mirroring. For example, although I might have interviewed someone about their experience of depression they may not be fully aware of all the factors that influence their experience – early life experiences, family beliefs, cultural expectations, the history of the concept itself (e.g., is it entirely synonymous with the ancient humoral notion of melancholia?). As a result, then, often our data will not be able to tell us 'directly and explicitly, what it might be (historically, for example, or politically), that drives, shapes and maintains these structures and practices' (Willig, in press) and so critical realists argue that we need to go beyond the text and draw on other evidence, perhaps from other disciplines. A number of psychotherapies could be located in this grouping including cognitive behaviour therapy and some forms of family therapy (e.g., structural and behavioural). For an example of how a critical realist position can inform the conceptualization of depression see Pilgrim and Bentall (1999). Dorling and Simpson (1999) gather together a range of work that could be termed critical realist. Thematic analysis and more realist forms of grounded theory could also be located here.

Phenomenology

Phenomenologists are interested in the nature of subjective experience from the perspective of research participants themselves. As a result, this is the framework that most often appeals to psychotherapeutically inclined researchers because their work is often focused on how a client subjectively experiences the world. There is less of a concern with whether what a person says – for example, about the past – is factually accurate. Rather, the focus is on understanding the past from the participant's perspective. Because of this, phenomenology is not at the direct realist end of the spectrum. However, it is equally not a relativist approach in that it is assumed there is some correspondence between what a person says and their subjective experience (although this might also be influenced by how much rapport the participant felt with the researcher and so on). For this reason it is often located roughly in the middle of the realism–relativism axis when it is represented in diagrammatic form. However, this axis privileges a method's stance on the status of 'external reality' but as this tends not to be a major concern for phenomenological traditions it is not easy to place on the continuum. Often, as a result, phenomenology is placed in the middle of the continuum but I think this is misleading rather than illuminating.

The humanistic psychotherapies could be located in this grouping as would Interpretative Phenomenological Analysis (IPA) and existentialist-informed phenomenology (see Chapters 8 and 9). There are two broad approaches to phenomenological research: descriptive and interpretative.

Descriptive phenomenology   Descriptive phenomenologists try to avoid imposing the researcher's categories or theories. Rather, the aim is to capture the essence of a participant's subjective experience in their own terms, delineating key elements and using the participant's terminology.

Interpretative phenomenology   Many phenomenologists wish to go beyond the text and, instead, to interpret the experience and so render it more meaningful. Larkin *et al.* (2006) and Chapter 8 suggest that this process of interpretation places a participant's account in a broader social, cultural and theoretical context. It is one of the tenets of IPA that the focus on interpretation foregrounds the interpretative role of the researcher.

Social constructionism

Social constructionist researchers are less focused on phenomena in themselves and are more interested in how the phenomena are seen. They are thus interested in how knowledge is generated – hence the focus on *construction* (Gergen, 1985). This generation is viewed as a primarily social process. Social constructionist are sceptical of the universal knowledge claims characteristic of direct realists, particularly in the social sciences, preferring more local and provisional claims. They question everyday taken-for-granted assumptions, arguing that these need to be seen in their social, historical and cultural context. Social constructionists are also interested in how some claims about reality are seen as having more validity than others. Because claims about knowledge are made through language, a study of how language is used is often a key focus in social constructionist work. Social constructionists differ from phenomenologists in that they do not see descriptions of experiences as windows onto a person's thoughts and feelings – rather, they view these as accounts that might be serving a range of interpersonal and societal functions. Moreover, they would see 'thoughts' and 'feelings' as concepts worthy of study in their own right – for example, they tell us about the ways in which socially and culturally available ways of talking about subjective experience are often dualistic and atomistic. Indeed, the *social* in social constructionism refers to the manner in which what is experienced by the individual is experienced through culturally shared categories of meaning – thus, the social constructionist project is critical of individualistic and intra-psychic approaches in the social sciences. Within psychology, the field of discursive psychology has attempted to take common psychological concepts like attitudes and reconceptualize them in a non-cognitive manner (e.g., Edwards & Potter, 1992). Willig (in press) characterizes the social constructionist researcher's role as that of an architect, interested both in how knowledge is created about the world and from what (cultural) resources and materials. They are interested in interrogating the implicit assumptions in texts that we normally take for granted, what the French literary theorist Jacques Derrida called 'deconstruction' (Derrida, 1967/1998).

Social constructionism is most associated with research methods that focus on language and the cultural and social availability of ways of seeing and talking about the world like discourse analysis and some Q methodology researchers (Curt, 1994; see also Chapter 14). More social constructionist versions of grounded theory would also be located here (see Chapter 10).

Sometimes, critics accuse social constructionist researchers of saying that phenomena such as psychological distress are '*just* social constructions' – the use of the word 'just' in these contexts adds to an impression that social constructionists deny that things like distress exists. This is not true – drawing attention to the fact that the way we conceive distress has changed throughout history and varies from place to place is not the same as saying it does not exist and that people do not experience it.

One important confusion to clear up is the difference between constructivism and social constructionism. Constructivism is a word best avoided by social constructionist researchers for a number of reasons, not least because it has a variety of technical meanings within other domains (e.g., perceptual and developmental psychology). It is also a well-established approach to therapy in the form of Personal Construct Theory (Kelly, 1955). Whilst constructivists acknowledge that individuals construct their own perceptions of the world, social constructionists go one step further, arguing that those individual constructions are developed in a social world where, moreover, different constructions have different social power. As a result, constructivism is not located at the relativist end of the realism–relativism spectrum. Confusingly, a number of authors use the term 'constructivism' or 'social constructivism' rather than 'social constructionism'. The more individualistic constructivist approach has influenced not only personal construct theory, but also a wide range of psychotherapies including cognitive behaviour therapy (Neimeyer, 1999). Social constructionism – which can be seen as the incorporation of many of the ideas associated with post-structualism and post-modernism (Harper & Spellman, 2006) – has had an influence on narrative and post-Milan family therapists and Lacanian psychoanalysis.

Social constructionism is relativist in a number of ways: its scepticism about a direct relationship between accounts and reality, and its assumption that we do not make direct contact with the world but, rather, our experience of it is mediated through culturally shared concepts – in other words, that language shapes our experience of reality. However, as Willig (in press) acknowledges, not all social constructionist researchers would describe themselves as relativists. Indeed, over the years commentators have identified two versions of social constructionism. One is described as a 'weak' or 'moderate' variant – which I term here as more critical realist (because this epistemological framework is often referred to by proponents). The other variant is described as 'strong' or 'radical' (although Smail, 2004, refers to it as 'naïve social constructionism', nicely mirroring the term 'naïve realism'). Here I will refer to it as the more relativist version because, again, this is the framework to which proponents tend to appeal. There is much debate within the broadly social constructionist community and Parker (1998) and Nightingale and Cromby (1999) are a good place to start in understanding the key issues.

Relativist social constructionism   Researchers adopting a more relativistic social constructionist perspective (or a 'radical constructionist' position) take the position that it is not possible to make comments about the nature of reality as we cannot be in direct contact with it. Instead, they argue, we should focus on what we can have contact with – what people say. In other words, one should not go beyond the text in order to interpret it. They treat the things that people say not as a window onto something else but as things worthy of study in and of themselves. A relativist position also means that there is no expectation that different researchers will see the same things in data – indeed, multiple interpretations or readings are to be expected.

A common misconception is that relativist researchers are relativist about everything and thus nihilistic. However, this is inaccurate – these researchers are usually only *epistemologically* or *methodologically* relativist, they are not necessarily *ontologically* relativist. In other words, they are relativist about what we can know about the world but they are not relativist about whether there is a world at all. An ontologically relativist claim would be that I do not know if there is a world or, indeed, that there are many worlds. However, an epistemological relativist goes about their life in the same way as everyone else, treating the world as if it exists. They simply claim that the focus of research should be on what is actually available to us (e.g., transcripts of talk) rather than abstract entities (like thoughts or feelings) which we can reach only via an inferential leap (Potter, 1996). However, as Hacking (2000) notes, many researchers do not make these somewhat subtle differentiations and some constructionist writers appear to conflate epistemological and ontological relativism. Another misapprehension is that epistemologically relativist social constructionists are moral relativists. However, simply noting there are different interpretations of data does not necessarily mean one is arguing that they are all equally as good from an ethical standpoint. Some epistemological relativists argue that relativism is consistent with a variety of ethical and political commitments (e.g., Curt, 1994; Hepburn, 2000; Shakespeare, 1998). Researchers using the variant of discourse analysis termed discursive psychology adopt a methodological relativism (Edwards & Potter, 1992; Hepburn & Wiggins, 2007; Potter, 2003).

Critical realist social constructionism   Researchers adopting this position (or a 'moderate constructionist' or critical theory approach) take the position that, alongside an awareness of the importance of studying qualitative data in detail, it is also important to go beyond the text in order to add a further layer of interpretation – by setting what is said in a broader historical, cultural and social context. These researchers, then, make certain ontological claims about pre-existing material practices which can influence discourse and thus they draw on some arguments similar to those of the critical realists noted in the realism section, whilst also drawing on social constructionist ideas. This grouping could be said to be ontologically realist but epistemologically relativist. Some researchers in this tradition use Foucauldian approaches to discourse analysis (see Arribas-Ayllon & Walkderdine, 2008; Parker, 1992, 2005).

Willig (in press) notes that critical realist constructionists are 'concerned with the ways in which available discourses can constrain and limit what can be said or done within particular contexts'. For example, how might the availability of things like childcare and employment affect the ways in which women talk about motherhood (Sims-Schouten *et al.*, 2007)? However, such readings can be heavily contested (see Speer, 2007, and the response by Riley *et al.*, 2007).

There have been vigorous debates between researchers from these two social constructionist groupings. Epistemologically relativist scholars argue that an ontological realism and epistemological relativism leads to inconsistency and a selective relativism in that the foundations of knowledge claims are only selectively being challenged. Problematizing some phenomena in an analysis whilst leaving others unproblematized has been termed 'ontological gerrymandering' (Woolgar & Pawluch, 1985) – referring to the practice of redrawing electoral boundaries in favour of a party or politician and so stacking the cards against other candidates. The reasons against seeing some phenomena (e.g., death) as constructed is said to be defended through the use of 'bottom line arguments' (Edwards *et al.*, 1995). Critical realists worry that the relativist position could lead to a political and moral relativism and that a failure to go beyond the text might mean that important issues like embodiment and subjectivity cannot be fully researched (Nightingale & Cromby, 1999; Gill, 1995; Parker, 1998; Velody & Williams, 1998).

Increasingly, some researchers have begun using a variety of methods simultaneously. When considering mixing quantitative and qualitative methods in this way it is essential to ensure there is epistemological consistency (see Box 7.3).

Box 7.3 Methodological Pluralism in Qualitative Research: 'Mixing' Methods

There are a number of different ways in which methods can be combined: using different kinds of qualitative data (e.g., naturalistic recordings plus interviews) but then analysing them within the same qualitative method of analysis; using different qualitative methods of analysis to analyse either one or a number of types of qualitative data; and combining both quantitative and qualitative data and methods of analysis.

Researchers may want to use more than one approach for a number of reasons. Because each method has its strengths and weaknesses, there is an argument that each method will be able to illuminate another layer of the topic. Another reason for mixing methods may relate to what data are most likely to persuade the intended audience. A full discussion of the issues involved in using different methods is beyond the scope of this chapter and book, but further discussion of some of the theoretical and practical issues involved can be seen in: Bryman (2006); Greene *et al.* (1989); Madill and Gough (2008); Todd *et al.* (2004); and Yardley and Bishop (2007). One of the dangers in mixing methods is that important differences in the epistemological assumptions of methods may not be considered (Madill & Gough, 2008).

Combining quantitative and qualitative methods

Here the strengths of qualitative research are combined with the ability of quantitative methods to investigate larger numbers of people, enabling statistical analysis. However, as noted earlier, this needs to occur within a coherent epistemology – for example, combining realist quantitative methods with more relativist qualitative methods may require a philosophically challenging rationale. Critical realism is a framework that could accommodate certain kinds of quantitative and qualitative research. When those influenced by post-structuralist and critical realist ideas use quantitative research, however, they adopt what Parker (1999) terms 'embedded objectivity' – in other words, they use it in a manner that is mindful of the status of numbers (Harré & Crystal, 2004):

(Continued)

Box 7.3 (*Cont'd*)

[T]here is no reason why qualitative research cannot work with figures, with records of observations, or with statistics as long as it is able to keep in mind that such data does not speak directly to us about facts 'out there' that are separate from us. Every bit of 'data' in research is itself a representation of the world suffused with interpretative work, and when we read the data we produce another layer of interpretations, another web of preconceptions and theoretical assumptions. Numeric data can help us to structure a mass of otherwise incomprehensible and overwhelming material, and statistical techniques can be very useful here, but our interpretations are also part of the picture, and so these interpretations need to be attended to (Parker, 1999, pp. 83–84).

Some psychotherapy and mental health training programmes promote the use of both quantitative and qualitative research methods. As I have noted, whilst this can work where the methods share epistemological assumptions it is impossible if they do not. Sometimes this approach is suggested for inappropriate reasons – supervisors might fear that a solely qualitative study will not be sufficient for postgraduate work – it is hoped that the range of work cited in the current volume will persuade them otherwise. Students in such situations need to cite the extant literature to not only demonstrate how inappropriate such demands are but, also find other ways of addressing what may be legitimate underlying concerns.

Using different qualitative methods

In Box 7.2 we saw how the same method could be used from different epistemological standpoints. However, recently researchers have used different qualitative methods to illuminate different aspects of the same data set – what some have termed a pluralistic approach to qualitative research (Frost, 2008). Thus, Wilkinson (2000) has compared the different analyses that can be developed in relation to women talking about breast cancer when using content analysis, a biographical approach and discourse analysis. Burck (2005) and Starks and Brown Trinidad (2007) use a similar approach in showing how different methods can illuminate different aspects of a topic. Focusing on the topic of delusions, Harper (2008) identifies the range of questions that have been asked by different methods drawing on different epistemological frameworks in relation to the topic of 'delusions'.

When you read the chapters in the next section, you can refer back to this discussion to see how that method can be located in these traditions. You will then be able to consider whether the claims and assumptions made within those traditions are ones that you wish to – and will have the data to – make. When using a method, it may be a useful (if not essential) exercise to make the assumptions underlying the method – and thus any claims generated using it – explicit. Doing so will enable you to consider carefully the suitability of all aspects of your proposed study and to choose appropriate criteria for evaluating the quality of your study (see Chapter 16). It is hoped that this chapter has helped to begin to demystify what is meant by epistemology and emphasized the importance of being able to demonstrate a clear rationale for the choice of a particular method.

References

Arribas-Ayllon, M. & Walkerdone, V. (2008). Foucauldian discourse analysis. In C. Willig & W. Stainton Rogers (Eds.) *The Sage handbook of qualitative research methods in psychology*. London: Sage.

Bryman, A. (2006). Integrating quantitative and qualitative research: How is it done? *Qualitative Research, 6*, 97–113.

Burck, C. (2005). Comparing qualitative research methodologies for systemic research: The use of grounded theory, discourse analysis and narrative analysis. *Journal of Family Therapy, 27*, 237–262.

Curt, B.C. (1994). *Textuality and tectonics: Troubling social and psychological science*. Buckingham: Open University Press.

Derrida, J. (1967/1998). *Of grammatology*. Translated by G.C. Spivak (Corrected Edition). Baltimore, MA: Johns Hopkins University Press.

Dorling, D. & Simpson, L. (Eds.) (1999). *Statistics in society: The arithmetic of politics*. London: Arnold.

Edwards, D., Ashmore, M. & Potter, J. (1995). Death and furniture: The rhetoric, politics and theology of bottom line arguments against relativism. *History of the Human Sciences, 8*, 25–49.

Edwards, D. & Potter, J. (1992). *Discursive psychology*. London: Sage.

Frost, N.A. (2008). Pluralism in qualitative research: Emerging findings from a study using mixed qualitative methods. *BPS Qualitative Methods in Psychology Section Newsletter*, October, 16–21.

Gergen, K.J. (1985). The social constructionist movement in modern psychology. *American Psychologist, 40*, 266–275.

Gill, R. (1995). Relativism, reflexivity and politics: Interrogating discourse analysis from a feminist perspective. In S. Wilkinson & C. Kitzinger (Eds.) *Feminism and discourse*. London: Sage.

Greene, J., Caracelli, V. & Graham, W. (1989). Toward a conceptual framework for mixed-method evaluation designs. *Educational Evaluation and Policy Analysis, 11*, 255–274.

Guba, E.G. & Lincoln, Y.S. (1994). Competing paradigms in qualitative research. In N.K. Denzin & Y.S. Lincoln (Eds.) *Handbook of qualitative research*. Thousand Oaks, CA: Sage.

Hacking, I. (2000). *The social construction of what?* London: Harvard University Press.

Harper, D. (2008). Clinical psychology. In C. Willig & W. Stainton Rogers (Eds.) *The Sage handbook of qualitative research methods in psychology*. London: Sage.

Harper, D. & Spellman, D. (2006). Telling a different story: Social constructionism and formulation. In L. Johnstone & R. Dallos (Eds.) *Formulation in psychology and psychotherapy: Making sense of people's problems*. London: Brunner-Routledge.

Harré, R. & Crystal, D. (2004). Discursive analysis and the interpretation of statistics. In Todd, Z., Nerlich, B., McKeown, S. & Clarke, D.D. (Eds.) *Mixing methods in psychology: The integration of qualitative and quantitative methods in theory and practice.* Hove: Psychology Press.

Hepburn, A. (2000). On the alleged incompatibility between feminism and relativism. *Feminism and Psychology, 10,* 91–106.

Hepburn, A. & Wiggins, S. (Eds.) (2007). *Discursive research in practice: New approaches to psychology and interaction.* Cambridge: Cambridge University Press.

Kelly, G. (1955) *The psychology of personal constructs.* New York: W.W. Norton.

Larkin, M., Watts, S. & Clifton, E. (2006). Giving voice and making sense in interpretative phenomenological analysis. *Qualitative Research in Psychology, 3,* 102–120.

Light, D. (1980). *Becoming psychiatrists: The professional transformation of self.* London: Norton.

Madill, A. & Gough, B. (2008). Qualitative research and its place in psychological science. *Psychological Methods, 13,* 254–271.

Madill, A., Jordan, A. & Shirley, C. (2000). Objectivity and reliability in qualitative analysis: Realist, contextualist and radical constructionist epistemologies. *British Journal of Psychology, 91,* 1–20.

Miller, E. (1999). Positivism and clinical psychology. *Clinical Psychology & Psychotherapy, 6,* 1–6.

Neimeyer, R.A. (1999) *Constructions of disorder: Meaning-making frameworks for psychotherapy.* Washington, D.C.: American Psychological Association.

Nightingale, D.J. & Cromby, J. (Eds.) (1999). *Social constructionist psychology: A critical analysis of theory and practice.* Buckingham: Open University Press.

Orne, M.T. (1962). On the social psychology of the psychological experiment: With particular reference to demand characteristics and their implications. *American Psychologist, 17,* 776–783.

Parker, I. (1992). *Discourse dynamics: Critical analysis for social and individual psychology.* London: Routledge.

Parker, I. (Ed.) (1998). *Social constructionism, discourse and realism.* London: Sage.

Parker, I. (1999). Qualitative data and the subjectivity of 'objective' facts, In D. Dorling & L. Simpson (Eds.) *Statistics in society: The arithmetic of politics.* London: Arnold.

Parker, I. (2005). *Qualitative psychology: Introducing radical research.* Maidenhead: Open University Press.

Pilgrim, D. & Bentall, R.P. (1999). The medicalisation of misery: A critical realist analysis of the concept of depression. *Journal of Mental Health, 8,* 261–274.

Potter, J. (1996). *Representing reality: Discourse, rhetoric and social construction.* London: Sage.

Potter, J. (2003). Discourse analysis and discursive psychology. In P.M. Camic, J.E. Rhodes & L. Yardley (Eds.) *Qualitative research in psychology: Expanding perspectives in methodology and design.* Washington: American Psychological Association.

Priebe, S. & Slade, M. (2006). Research production and consumption. In M. Slade & S. Priebe (Eds.) *Choosing methods in mental health research.* London: Routledge.

Riley, S.C.E., Sims-Schouten, W. & Willig, C. (2007). The case for critical realist discourse analysis as a viable method in discursive work. *Theory and Psychology, 17,* 137–145.

Shadish, W.R. (1995). Philosophy of science and the quantitative-qualitative debates: Thirteen common errors. *Evaluation and Programme Planning, 18,* 63–75.

Shakespeare, T. (1998). Social constructionism as a political strategy. In I. Velody & R. Williams (Eds.) *The politics of constructionism.* London: Sage.

Sims-Schouten, W., Riley, S.C.E. & Willig, C. (2007). Critical realism in discourse analysis: A presentation of a systematic method of analysis using women's talk of motherhood, childcare and female employment as an example. *Theory and Psychology, 17*, 101–124.

Speer, S.A. (2007). On recruiting conversation analysis for critical realist purposes. *Theory and Psychology, 17*, 125–135.

Slade, M. & Priebe, S. (2006). Who is research for? In M. Slade & S. Priebe (Eds.) *Choosing methods in mental health research.* London: Routledge.

Smail, D. (2004). Psychotherapy and the making of subjectivity. In P. Gordon & R. Mayo (Eds.) *Between psychotherapy and philosophy.* London and Philadelphia: Whurr.

Starks, H. & Brown Trinidad, S. (2007). Choose your method: A comparison of phenomenology, discourse analysis, and grounded theory. *Qualitative Health Research, 17*, 1372–1380.

Todd, Z., Nerlich, B., McKeown, S. & Clarke, D.D. (Eds.) (2004). *Mixing methods in psychology: The integration of qualitative and quantitative methods in theory and practice.* Hove: Psychology Press.

Velody, I. & Williams, R. (Eds.) (1998). *The politics of constructionism.* London: Sage.

Wilkinson, S. (2000). Women with breast cancer talking causes: Comparing content, biographical and discursive analyses. *Feminism and Psychology, 10*, 431–460.

Willig, C. (in press). Perspectives on the epistemological bases for qualitative research. In H. Cooper (Ed.) *The handbook of research methods in psychology.* Washington, D.C.: American Psychological Association.

Woolgar, S. & Pawluch, D. (1985). Ontological gerrymandering. *Social Problems, 32*, 214–227.

Yardley, L. & Bishop, F. (2007). Mixing qualitative and quantitative methods: A pragmatic approach. In C. Willig & W. Stainton-Rogers (Eds.) *Handbook of qualitative research methods in psychology.* London: Sage.

Further reading and a useful website

Guba, E.G. & Lincoln, Y.S. (1994). Competing paradigms in qualitative research. In N.K. Denzin & Y.S. Lincoln (Eds.) *Handbook of qualitative research.* Thousand Oaks, CA: Sage.

Priebe, S. & Slade, M. (2006). Research production and consumption. In M. Slade & S. Priebe (Eds.) *Choosing methods in mental health research.* London: Routledge.

Willig, C. (in press). Perspectives on the epistemological bases for qualitative research. In H. Cooper (Ed.) *The handbook of research methods in psychology.* Washington, DC: American Psychological Association.

Online resource for choosing between methods hosted by Huddersfield University: http://onlineqda.hud.ac.uk/methodologies.php.

Part II

Methods

8

Interpretative Phenomenological Analysis in Mental Health and Psychotherapy Research

Michael Larkin and Andrew R. Thompson

Description of the Method

Interpretative Phenomenological Analysis (IPA; Smith *et al.*, 2009) is an approach to qualitative analysis with a particularly psychological interest in how people make sense of their experience. IPA requires the researcher to collect detailed, reflective, first-person accounts from research participants. It provides an established, phenomenologically focused approach to the interpretation of these accounts. It draws on a similar body of philosophical influences to the existential approach outlined in the next chapter, but the analytic processes and outcomes are rather different.

The outcome of a successful IPA study is likely to include an element of '*giving voice*' (capturing and reflecting upon the principal claims and concerns of the research participants) and '*making sense*' (offering an interpretation of this material, which is grounded in the accounts, but may use psychological concepts to extend beyond them; see e.g., Larkin *et al.*, 2006). IPA is a relatively accessible qualitative approach – and there are lots of published examples and methods articles to draw upon – but striking the right balance between these two key components takes considerable time and effort. This is often best conducted in the context of supervision and peer support, which can facilitate the development and discussion of these elements.

Qualitative Research Methods in Mental Health and Psychotherapy: A Guide for Students and Practitioners, First Edition.
Edited by D. Harper and A.R. Thompson.
© 2012 John Wiley & Sons, Ltd. Published 2012 by John Wiley & Sons, Ltd.

Origins and Influences

Idiography and hermeneutic phenomenology and are the key conceptual touchstones for IPA. As with other qualitative approaches, IPA is concerned with meaning and processes, rather than with events and their causes. In the case of IPA, meaning-making is conceptualized at the level of the *person-in-context*. This means that we focus first on the meaning of an experience (e.g., an event, process or relationship) to a given participant, and recognize its significance *for that participant*. In this way, IPA has a commitment to an *idiographic* level of analysis – which implies a focus on the particular, rather than the general. This connects closely with IPA's engagement with hermeneutic phenomenology.

Phenomenology is the philosophical study of 'Being' (i.e., of existence and experience). It is often understood to have two important historical phases: the transcendental, and the hermeneutic or existential. Transcendental phenomenology – from Husserl – strives to identify the essential core structures of a given experience (through a process of methodological 'reductions'). For Husserl, phenomenology was about identifying and suspending our assumptions ('bracketing' off culture, context, history, etc.) in order to get at the universal essence of a given phenomenon, as it presents itself to consciousness. His phenomenology aimed to *transcend* our everyday assumptions. These ideas have been particularly influential on the more 'descriptive' forms of phenomenological psychology (see e.g., Giorgi & Giorgi, 2003).

IPA does not aim for transcendent knowledge. Instead, it draws upon the later re-readings of phenomenology developed by Husserl's successors. These writers – notably Heidegger and Merleau-Ponty – suggest that we can never make Husserl's 'reduction' to the abstract, because our observations are always made from *somewhere*. For Heidegger, persons (*Dasein*, 'there-being') are inextricably involved in the world, and in relationships with others. For Merleau-Ponty, persons are always embodied too. These facts shape our perception of the world. Such strong emphases on the *worldly* and *embodied* nature of our existence suggest that phenomenological inquiry is a *situated* enterprise. This position is often called *hermeneutic phenomenology*, to emphasize that, while phenomenology might be descriptive in its inclination, it can only ever be *interpretative* in its implementation.

Epistemological Assumptions

IPA has an interpretative (aka hermeneutic) phenomenological epistemology. We are interested in understanding a person's *relatedness* to the world (and to the things in it which matter to them) through the meanings that they make. Thus, IPA proceeds on the following assumptions:

- An understanding of the world requires an understanding of experience.
- IPA researchers elicit and engage with the personal accounts of other people who are 'always-already' immersed in a linguistic, relational, cultural and physical world.
- We therefore need to take an idiographic approach to our work, in order to facilitate a detailed focus on the *particular*.

- Researchers do not access experience directly from these accounts, but through a process of intersubjective meaning-making.
- In order to engage with other people's experience, researchers need to be able to identify and reflect upon their own experiences and assumptions.
- We cannot escape interpretation at any stage, but we can reflect upon our role in producing these interpretations, and we can maintain a commitment to grounding them in our participants' views.

What Kind of Research Questions Suit IPA?

The topic should be something that *matters* to the participants, who are usually selected purposively, precisely because they can offer a valuable perspective on the topic at hand. This means that samples in IPA are usually reasonably homogeneous; participants tend to have *understanding* of the topic at hand. Typically, this understanding is experiential – IPA is not usually used to study people's attitudes to issues that are of no direct relevance to their lives.

IPA requires open research questions, focused on the experiences, and/or understandings, of particular people in a particular context. The intent is exploratory rather than explanatory; for example:

- How do people seeking support through self-help programmes make sense of their experiences of addiction and recovery (e.g., Larkin, 2001)?
- How do members of a community mental health team communicate and make sense of complex clinical presentations like personality disorder (e.g., Donnison *et al.*, 2009)?

These are first-tier questions. All IPA projects have these. Some projects will also have second-tier questions. These may be used to engage with theory. IPA does not test hypotheses, and is not usually used to build theory per se – but its analytic outcomes can be used to open up a dialogue with extant theory. It is useful to have a few more refined or theoretically informed questions, but to treat these as 'secondary' – because they can only be answered at the discussion stage. For example, we might have a primary research question which is very open (such as 'How do people make sense of their treatment decisions?'). More pointed questions (such as 'How do accounts of the decision-making process relate to the model described in theory *Y*?') can be secondary.

What Kind of Data is Appropriate for IPA?

IPA usually requires a verbatim transcript of a first-person account, which has been generated by a research participant, usually in response to an invitation by a researcher. Most typically, this is in the form of a semi-structured, one-to-one interview (Smith *et al.*, 2009). Other forms of data that can sometimes be used for IPA include written accounts (Smith, 1999) and focus groups (Palmer *et al.*, 2010). In either case, the assumption is that the researcher will aim to take a role that is as neutral and facilitative, and provides participants with an opportunity to tell their story. There is a recognition that one cannot be truly neutral, and that the interview situation comes with certain expectations. However, the researcher is aiming to capture an account that is rich, detailed and reflective. An IPA interview is not about collecting facts, it is about exploring meanings.

IPA studies require small sample sizes. It is the quality, rather than the quantity of data that permits insightful analyses to be developed. Appropriate numbers of participants will vary according to the aims, level and context of the research, and the time and resources of the researcher (for more detail see Smith *et al.*, 2009; Thompson *et al.*, in press). IPA also lends itself to single case study analysis – although this may be more suited to more experienced researchers.

Thinking about depth or range may be more helpful than thinking about numbers. For example, it can be helpful to interview participants twice, or to use diaries or other additional tools to facilitate understanding between the researcher and participant. Expanding the design, to include interviews with related respondents can also be helpful.

How Can IPA Involve Service Users and People from the Research Population Under Study?

There are different levels and approaches to involvement. So far, few IPA studies have addressed the nuances of this, but it is not unusual for the research population to be involved in the early stages of an IPA project, in the 'piloting' of interview schedules, or in assisting the research team to consider ethical issues. Only one IPA mental health study to date has been commissioned and conducted by service users. Pitt *et al.* (2007) describe how a committee of service users had significant role in planning their study, and how service user researchers then led the data collection, analysis and write-up.

Few studies have been fully participatory. One exception is Martindale *et al.*'s (2009) study, which sought to explore experiences of confidentiality and consent for users of clinical psychology services. Their data were collected by service user researchers, and the analysis was conducted jointly by a service user researcher and a psychologist. The authors discuss some of the complexities involved in conducting their research, openly acknowledging that it led to 'lengthy debates' (Martindale *et al.*, 2009, p. 366).

A Step-by-Step Approach to Using IPA

When you interpret qualitative data, you aim to develop an *organized, detailed, plausible* and *transparent* account of the *meaning* of the data. To do this, first, you need to identify *patterns of meaning* in the data. In IPA, these patterns are usually called '*themes*' and the themes are usually drawn from detailed, line-by-line commentary on the data, called '*codes*'. Eventually, you will want to be able to draw your themes together in to some kind of structure (this might be a table, a hierarchy, like a family tree, or a more circular diagrammatic representation) so that you can present your reader with an overview of the analysis. Secondly, you will need to produce a narrative account of this structure for the analysis section of your report. You will want to be able to steer the reader through your analytic work, giving examples of the things that matter to participants, highlighting your interpretations of their accounts, and taking time to explore any data that do not fit the prevailing patterns.

Remember in IPA we are interested in identifying what *matters* to participants, and then exploring what these things *mean* to participants. Once we have some understanding of this, we can develop an interpretative synthesis of the analytic work. The process for reaching that point in IPA is *iterative* and *inductive*, cycling and recycling through the strategies in Box 8.1.

Box 8.1 Analytic Process in IPA

- IPA analysis begins at the level of the individual case, with close, line-by-line analysis (i.e., *coding*) of the experiential claims, concerns and understandings of each participant (see e.g., Larkin *et al.*, 2006).
- Identification of the emergent patterns (i.e., *themes*) within this experiential material emphasizing both convergence and divergence, commonality and nuance (see e.g., Eatough & Smith, 2008); usually first for single cases, and then subsequently across multiple cases.
- Development of a 'dialogue' between the researchers, their coded data and their psychological knowledge, about what it might *mean* for participants to have these concerns in this context (see e.g., Larkin *et al.*, 2006; Smith, 2004), leading in turn to the development of a more *interpretative account.*
- Development of a *structure*, frame or gestalt which illustrates the relationships between themes.
- *Organization* of all of this material in a format that allows for coded data to be traced right through the analysis – from initial codes on the transcript, through initial clustering and thematic development, into the final structure of themes.
- Use of *supervision or collaboration, to audit,* to help test and develop the coherence and plausibility of the interpretation and explore reflexivity.
- Development of a *narrative*, evidenced by detailed commentary on data extracts, which takes the reader through this interpretation, usually theme-by-theme, and often supported by some form of *visual guide* (simple heuristic diagram or table).
- *Reflection* on one's own perceptions, conceptions and processes should occur throughout the process and is usually captured in a systematic fashion by keeping a reflexive journal (see e.g., Smith, 2007).

List from Smith *et al.*, 2009, p. 79–80; our italics.

Within these strategies, there is considerable room for manoeuvre. The epistemological focus of IPA can be implemented with flexibility, and other authors offer additional guidance on further analytic strategies (e.g., Eatough & Smith, 2008; Smith *et al.*, 2009).

In the next section, we describe some of the key features in more depth. In our experience, reflection, which is the last element listed above, makes a good place to start and finish.

Reflection on one's own preconceptions through 'free' or 'open' coding

It can be helpful to start by working with a licence to be wrong, presumptive, wayward, biased, creative, self-absorbed and unsystematic. Take a clean copy of the transcript, read through it a couple of times and write all over it. You can write anything: your own emotional reactions to the participant and their story, as you now recall the interview; initial ideas about potential themes; metaphors and imagery that strike you as particularly powerful; psychological concepts that seem to leap out at you from the data, as though calling directly on your theoretical knowledge.

This 'free coding' is partly about getting your initial ideas down, so that you can then proceed with a more systematic and consistent focus (below). It is also partly about identifying and considering the influence of your preconceptions. We cannot seal these off in a vacuum, but we can aim to be open-minded, to reveal our biases where possible and to minimize their impact. This is an ongoing reflexive process, which runs right through the life of a project. It can help to keep a reflexive journal detailing the process. It is also helpful to talk through examples of your free coding and personal reflections in supervision or with peer researchers, as preparation for more systematic coding.

The close, line-by-line analysis (i.e., coding) of the experiential claims, concerns and understandings of each participant – 'phenomenological' coding

Remaining at the level of the first case, now set aside your free-coded transcript and start fresh, with a clean copy. Your core analysis will be developed through the detailed, line-by-line annotation of the transcript. In particular, you will find it helpful to identify 'objects of concern' (anything that matters to the participants; e.g., events, relationships, values, etc.) and then to look for 'experiential claims' (these are linguistic and narrative clues as to the *meaning* of those objects). For example, consider this short extract from an interview with a male stroke survivor.

There is clearly something that *matters* to the participant in this short narrative, something that is 'annoying'. We might call it 'face', 'social standing' or, more generally, 'identity.' Its meaning – the experiential claim that underpins both the story and the thing exemplified – seems to have something to do with 'disempowerment' or 'invisibility'. The participant appears to feel that his identity – as an active able man who warrants recognition and attention from people that he knows, or from 'officials' – has been

Developing line-by-line coding, staying close to data; generating possible interpretations	Transcript excerpt	Checking/clarifying core content
(Something is) *annoying* • I don't go out much (*very occasionally*) • I have to use the wheelchair • '*The wife*' pushes me **(Loss of agency/mobility)** – *threat to masculinity?* • People we know . . . • Officials (important people?) . . . • . . . talk to my wife, *not to me* **(Loss of face/status)** – this is what's *annoying*	Well the annoying thing is, when I go out, very occasionally, it has to be in a wheelchair. Now, when the wife is pushing me, er, we may see someone that we know or possibly an official. That person talks to my wife rather than me'	*Object of concern:* Other people's lack of recognition of/respect for my status as a human being *Experiential claim:* This is 'annoying' (understate-ment?) **Spoiled identity?**

diminished, by the wheelchair, and possibly by the presence of his wife, pushing the wheelchair.

The process of identifying, and noting down these observations tends to involve some parallel processes. The analyst is developing line-by-line coding, and trying to stay close to the data, but will also be beginning to generate possible interpretations (see next subsection). As the level of annotation starts to 'thicken out', they may also be checking and clarifying the core experiential content of the work that they have completed so far. The cycle of engaging with the data should explore all possibilities in depth. It is important to record these codes, and to discuss and evaluate this work in supervision or with peer researchers, because it takes practice to develop rigour and sustain a consistent focus. Note that, as in the example above, you will also be generating some ideas about the data at this stage which may feel as though they are more explicitly 'interpretative', and which already seem to be stepping a little beyond the experiential claims and concerns which are your primary focus.

Identification of emerging themes

Once a transcript has been coded in detail, with a primary focus on the experiential content, it can be helpful to do some preliminary organizing and summarizing of the work completed so far. This is likely to happen, first of all, at the level of individual cases. It is therefore important that these initial case-level themes are captured in a flexible manner, because later on, when you proceed to looking at the data in a more 'cross-sectional' manner (i.e., once you begin to look for common themes *across* the cases), you will need to be able to spot potential connections across multiple levels of conceptualization.

Conducting some initial case-level work will help you to see the benefits of your efforts, in attending to the detail of the account, and will also give you a useful platform for further interpretative work with this transcript, and further integration across multiple transcripts at the next stage.

One useful way of doing this is to cluster the work that you have done around 'things that matter' (objects of concern) and the meanings that are attached to them (experiential claims). These will be quite small units of meaning – so there will be a lot of them at this stage. They should also be seen as tentative, emerging ideas – and so it may not be so helpful to give them specific titles, which might 'fix' their meaning a little too narrowly. Identifying 'bundles' of terms or phrases which capture the complexity of the content can be a better strategy – see Box 8.2 for an example.

Box 8.2 Keeping Track of the Emerging Themes

Diagnosis is . . .
1/41 – required as an end goal
2/16 – described as disreputable or sinful
2/24 – irrelevant, bears no relation to people's lives
2/32 – something that dictates treatment, removes thinking process, is functional but. . .
3/10 – insensitive/reductionist, might miss something meaningful
3/11 – leads to stigma, discrimination, exclusion
3/33 – outdated, does not view the person
4/35 – requires interpretation of experiences
7/32 – unavoidable if you know criteria (trapped by the knowledge?) but does not need to be stated
7/35 – something that patients must be protected from
9/10 – a careless, even aggressive, act
10/18 – polarized against meaning
10/24 – an easy way out, does not require thought
12/19 – 'by looking at symptoms you are missing the person' and that is more real/certain

These are all of the meanings attached by one participant to one object of concern (in this case 'diagnosis' – the participant is a psychiatrist). They are all identified by page and line number so that the context of these claims and concerns can easily be checked against any developing interpretations

- Diagnosis as a necessary functional tool/object
- A damaging object, to be avoided to minimize harm
- A blunt implement (lazy, careless, insensitive, outdated)
- Meaningless (to the patient and also polarized against meaningfulness)

This is the analyst's summarizing work which identifies the cluster of meanings that characterize the content, above

Example from De Boos (2008)

Development of a 'dialogue' between the researchers, their coded data and their psychological knowledge, about what it might mean for participants to have these concerns, in this context

Once you are happy that you have mapped out the 'phenomenological core' of the data in sufficient detail (probably for each of your transcripts), you will want to return to some of the more explicitly interpretative ideas that you have been documenting, and work on those. At this point, your analysis may start to develop a more speculative, questioning dimension. You will find that, as with the early stage of line-by-line coding, there are a number of parallel processes here, and that this work is closely linked with, and developed from, the work that you have already completed. For example, in the extract below, we can see several strategies illustrated in the interplay between the 'phenomenological coding' (on the left) and the more explicitly 'interpretative' coding (on the right). The participant is a woman in late middle-age, who takes part in bungee-jumping most weekends.

PROMPT: planning?	I: So are there specific things that you kind of plan to do when you do the jump? Do you (think R: There) are now, because I'm more into the serious stage of it now.	Offering *opportunity* to demonstrate planning (what does it mean to plan?)
• serious = • progression from earlier stages		
	I: Yeah.	*Activity has value, requires experience, skill and preparation – like a sport, not 'pure' hedonism?*
• experienced (quantity of jumps)	R: Where I've done, obviously, quite a number of jumps. I: Yeah.	
• plan	R: And we do plan the jump sometimes. I: Yeah.	*We:* This is a process shared with – and validated by – others
• somersaults, rolls *(versatility, variability, skill)*	R: You know like I'll do three somersaults, or three rolls or whatever. I: Yeah.	
• backwards, forwards	R: (pause) Or whether I'll get out backwards, forwards or/Yes, we do plan it more now, yes.	*Presents multiple opportunities for variability of experience to skilled jumper*
• PROMPT: satisfaction?	I: And is there added satisfaction in that [then, I R: Well there is, if you do a	
• good, splendid, lovely – 'like I did' – satisfied *(warm, gentle)*	really good jump and you've done some splendid somersaults, like I did one	Expression of agency and skills is rewarding in itself

	today that had some lovely	*Why so warm/gentle? (More*
• a good job (*performance, execution, achievement*) • if . . . a bad one (*not predictable*) • you just think (*acceptable*)	somersaults in it (pause) yes, you are satisfied when you've made a really good job of it. I: Yeah. R: And if you've done a bad one you just think, you know – '(*huf*) – that was a mess' – you know? (laughs) **Emily, bungee, lines 57–75**	*'flow' than 'buzz'?)* Experience is not entirely predictable – there are skills you can develop to allow you to maximize time, control the feeling, demonstrate experience But sometimes you just have to accept a 'bad one'

Here the analyst can be seen to be:

1. *Identifying cumulative patterns within transcripts* (e.g., Emily's use of the collective voice, '*We* do plan the jump'). Emily often speaks for her bungee-jumping community in the interview, and in other places she emphasizes the importance of the social support and the benefits of shared enterprise. When we see all of that information in one place, we begin to see a pattern for Emily, where *being part of a community* is a very positive aspect of bungee-jumping.

2. *Engaging with imagery and metaphor.* In this instance there is an underlying analogy between 'bungee-jumping' and 'sport' which connects various features of this extract (emphasizing skill, experience, performance) to features evident elsewhere in the interview (down-playing risk, emphasizing safety procedures and favourably comparing bungee-jumping with joyriding).

3. *Synthesizing or collapsing the first-order coding to develop more abstract categories.* When we consider the opportunities presented to Emily by the 'somersaults/rolls' and 'backwards/forwards' pairs, we gain some insight into the *multiple opportunities for varying one's experience* which are available to a the skilled jumper.

4. *Taking a more interrogative approach to the coding.* There may be aspects of the data that prompt us to ask questions. Why is Emily's language so strikingly warm and gentle ('good', 'splendid', 'lovely')? Perhaps it stands out for us because we are more accustomed to people drawing upon the prevailing language of 'risk' and 'adrenalin' to represent their experiences of activities like bungee-jumping.

5. *Opening some cautious dialogue with theory.* Emily's use of this counter-intuitive language, combined with the emphasis on performance and skill, are reminiscent of some of Csikszentmihalyi and Csikszentmihalyi's (1988) ideas about 'flow experiences' (the details of Csikszentmihalyi & Csikszentmihalyi's work are not that important here; it is simply that there is a resonance between an emerging interpretation and an existing psychological concept). Note that the theory is not being imported here to 'explain away' the data. It is being offered more cautiously, as a

concept that may prove to be useful at the discussion stage (i.e., it may be helpful to have 'flow' in mind as we try to understand Emily's point of view). This allows us to see the phenomenon from the perspective of conceptual resources which can lead us to a richer, more insightful and more psychological account.

6. *Identifying cumulative patterns across transcripts.* This particular study explored notions of 'risk' and 'reward' as they were understood by both bungee-jumpers and recreational Ecstasy-users (Larkin & Griffiths, 2004). When we paraphrase Emily's account here at an abstract level, we can see some potential commonalities between the accounts of the two groups. To paraphrase: this experience is not entirely predictable – but there are skills you can develop which will allow you to demonstrate your expertise and experience to others, and to maximize the time where you are able control the shift in your experience of yourself (this is when you are weightless, for the bungee-jumpers, and when you are 'up' for the drug-users) … but, despite all this, sometimes you just have to accept a 'bad one'.

These are not the only forms of interpretative work that may be used in IPA, but they are some of the key elements of most people's implementation of the approach. As we hope we have demonstrated, interpretative coding *should* develop from, or connect to, the core experiential material, but it need not be entirely constrained by it.

Note that, at some point during this stage of your analysis, you will be beginning to work across the data set, spotting connections between cases and identifying the concepts and labels for themes which capture what is important across the dataset as a whole. The next step, then, is to focus upon this more directly.

Development of a structure that illustrates the relationships between themes

As your interpretative ideas develop, you will start to spot the different ways in which your long, previously-collated set of emerging themes could be organized into a more economical and evocative pattern. This process requires considerable time, reflection and discussion before you settle on a solution that best represents the patterns of meaning in your data set, and accommodates the convergence and divergence within it. This can be done by way of cutting-and-pasting or computer software. Excerpts can then be arranged and rearranged, until their relationships with one another are adequately expressed by way of a visible structure. You should find that you benefit from having retained open and flexible labels for the emerging themes at the previous stages. Once again, there will be considerable iterative movement until you settle on labels. The most effective theme labels are usually those that clearly evoke the content of the material within them, *and* the meanings that are attached to that content by the participants.

This final structure might be hierarchical or it may be in the form of table, or circular account. Note that the resulting structure is not *explanatory* and is not a *model* of what is 'out there' (although it will be a representation of *your analysis* and may still share some similarities with the formulatory approach common to many psychological therapeutic approaches). Constructing this sort of heuristic should help you to understand and develop the relationships between themes. It should also be accessible to someone who does not know your data (see Table 8.1 for a fictional example, illustrating one theme from a study exploring experiences of hospitalization.

Quality Issues

IPA is interpretative, so some validation strategies, such as 'member-checking,' may be less appropriate than others. Member-checking may be appropriate for single case designs, where the interpretation offered can be traced back to one person's account. For designs with multiple participants, the combined effects of amalgamation of accounts, interpretation by the researcher and the passage of time, can make member-checking counter-productive. It is often preferable to use sample validation (people eligible to participate, but who did not), peer validation (fellow researchers) or audit. Whether you intend to use audit, or other processes of credibility checking, to test the coherence and plausibility of your analysis, a document such as in Table 8.1 is likely to have a key role in facilitating the process.

Smith (2010) has recently published a systematic review of IPA papers and described some of the general quality indicators that one might look for. We would also suggest that a 'good' piece of IPA research is likely to demonstrate most of the following features:

- Collecting appropriate data, from appropriately selected informants.
- Some degree of idiographic focus (attention to the particular) balanced against 'what is shared' within a sample.
- An analysis that:
  - transcends the structure of the data collection method (e.g., the schedule for a semi-structured interview)
  - focuses on 'how things are understood', rather than on 'what happened'
  - incorporates and balances phenomenological detail (where appropriate) and interpretative work (where appropriate) to develop a psychologically relevant account of the participants' 'engagement-in-the-world'.
- Appropriate use of triangulation (can be via methods, perspectives, data, analysts, fieldwork) or audit and/or credibility-checking (can be via respondents, supervisors, peers, parallel sample) to achieve trustworthiness.
- Appropriate use of extracts and commentary to achieve transparency (claims should usually be referenced to data; data should not usually be left to 'speak for themselves'; there should be substantive engagement with, and commentary on some longer extracts of data).
- Appropriate level of contextual detail – for the extracts, participants, researchers and study.
- Attention to process; including both analytic and reflexive components.
- Appropriate pitch and engagement with theory (in making sense of the analysis).

Table 8.1 Example of final structure showing one theme at the level of an across-transcripts analysis

Superordinate theme	Participants contributing to this theme	Subthemes	Participants contributing to this sub-theme	Key cross-references	Indicative quotes	Notes
Expecting and experiencing hospitals to be difficult places to be	All except Peter	Adapting to an alien environment (frightening, noisy, strange smell, maze-like, weird; a place for adults)	Sandi, Nick, Sasha, Ali, Ellen, Charlie	Sandi (L24, 75), Nick (L55, L120, L250), Sasha (L5, L10, L80, L200, L220), Ali (L23, L40, L48, L212), Ellen (L30, L42), Charlie (L8, L55)	'When we went to see the doctors we had to wait for a really really long time, and the telly was just showing – I don't know what rubbish – and the smell made me feel a bit sick' (Nick) 'Walking down the corridors is a bit like being lost underground or something' (Charlie)	Peter is a counter-case here, because his father is a nurse in the hospital where he will be treated; hospitals in general are relatively familiar to him, and he talks positively of going to visit 'Dad's work'
		Worrying about pain and/or intrusive interventions	Sandi, Nick, Sasha, Ali, Ellen, Charlie	Sandi (L32, 183), Nick (L26), Sasha (L47), Ali (L33, L90), Ellen (L101), Charlie (L19, L36, L305)	'I know I might have to have an injection, and I've had one before, but I don't remember it, so I am a bit worried about that' (Sasha)	Most of the participants had some concerns about this, largely in the short-term (i.e., what the doctors will do when I go to stay in the hospital)

- Engagement with other IPA work and/or phenomenological theory.
- Appropriate understanding and implementation of transferability issues.

How Might Studies Using This Method Relate to the Development of Mental Health Policy?

IPA studies can provide crucial insights into personal experiences and psychosocial processes. These insights can be valuable on a number of levels (Box 8.3). They may not tell us what causes x, or whether y works – but they can help us to understand what it is *like* to live with x, and *how y* works.

Box 8.3 IPA Research May Help Us To:

- Understand the experiences of particular groups of people
- Develop and evaluate services, therapeutic interventions, and so on
- Interpret the associative findings from conventional quantitative research
- Situate and understand people in their socio-cultural contexts
- Evaluate and reflect upon the role played by therapeutic, institutional and legislative cultures
- Re-evaluate existing theory

Future Directions

We hope this chapter has demonstrated how IPA can explore mental health issues. IPA studies have already made an important contribution to knowledge in the mental health field.

IPA researchers may wish to consider when and how to better involve service users. The balance between phenomenological and interpretative elements in IPA means that there will be some dilemmas involved in doing this, but IPA's overarching commitment to understanding experience means that these can be addressed. Good IPA often comes about as a joint venture.

Systemic or multi-perspectival designs offer another potentially fruitful future development of IPA in the field of mental health. Given that the needs of service users, carers, families and service providers are often overlapping but also quite distinct, designs that look at a phenomenon from a number of inter-related perspectives (e.g., foster carers, looked-after children and social workers; Rostill *et al.*, 2010) can offer powerful new insights.

Lastly, we would encourage people who wish to use IPA to be creative, and to think carefully about data collection, taking great care to engage with participants on terms that are amenable and meaningful to them, and giving careful consideration to the use of case study analysis, and to triangulation of data collection between interviews and other forms, such as diaries or group discussions.

References

Csikszentmihalyi, M. & Csikszentmihalyi, I.S. (1988). *Optimal experience: Psychological studies of flow in consciousness.* Cambridge, UK: Cambridge University Press.

De Boos, D. (2008). A qualitative exploration of the process of diagnosing black and minority ethnic men. Doctoral thesis, University of Birmingham.

Donnison, J., Thompson, A.R. & Turpin, G. (2009). A qualitative study of the conceptual models employed by community mental health team staff. *International Journal of Mental Health Nursing, 18,* 310–317.

Dreyfus, H. (2007). Philosophy 185: Heidegger's *Being and Time.* University of California, Berkeley. Webcasts available at: http://webcast.berkeley.edu/course_details.php?seriesid= 1906978475.

Eatough, V. & Smith, J.A. (2008). Interpretative phenomenological analysis. In C. Willig & W. Stainton Rogers (Eds.)*Handbook of qualitative psychology* (pp. 179–194). London: Sage.

Giorgi, A. & Giorgi, B. (2003). Phenomenology. In J.A. Smith (Ed.) *Qualitative psychology: A practical guide to research methods* (pp. 25–50). London: Sage.

Langridge, D. (2007). *Phenomenological psychology.* Harlow: Pearson.

Larkin, M. (2001). Understandings and experiences: A post-constructionist cultural psychology of addiction and recovery in the 12-step tradition. Doctoral dissertation, Nottingham Trent University, Nottingham, UK.

Larkin, M. & Griffiths, M.D. (2004). Dangerous sports and recreational drug-use: rationalizing and contextualizing risk. *Journal of Community and Applied Social Psychology, 14,* 215–232.

Larkin, M., Watts, S. & Clifton, E. (2006). Giving voice and making sense in Interpretative Phenomenological Analysis. *Qualitative Research in Psychology, 3,* 102–120.

Martindale, S.J., Chambers, E. & Thompson, A.R. (2009). Clinical psychology service users' experiences of confidentiality and informed consent: a qualitative analysis. *Psychology and Psychotherapy: Theory, Research and Practice, 82,* 355–368.

Moran, D. (2000). *Introduction to phenomenology.* London: Routledge.

Palmer, M., Larkin, M., De Visser, R. & Fadden, G. (2010). Developing an interpretative phenomenological approach to focus group data. *Qualitative Research in Psychology, 7,* 99–121.

Pitt, L., Kilbride, M., Nothard, S., Welford, M. & Morrison, A.P. (2007). Researching recovery from psychosis: A user-led project. *Psychiatric Bulletin, 31,* 55–60.

Rostill, H., Larkin, M., Toms, A. & Churchman, C. (2010). A shared experience of fragmentation: Making sense of foster placement breakdown. *Clinical Child Psychology and Psychiatry,* doi:10.1177/1359104509352894.

Smith, J.A. (1999). Towards a relational self: Social engagement during pregnancy and psychological preparation for motherhood. *British Journal of Social Psychology, 38,* 409–426.

Smith, J.A. (2004). Reflecting on the development of interpretative phenomenological analysis and its contribution to qualitative research in psychology. *Qualitative Research in Psychology, 1,* 39–54.

Smith, J.A. 2007). Hermeneutics, human sciences and health: linking theory and practice. *International Journal of Qualitative Studies on Health and Well-being, 2,* 3–11.

Smith, J.A. (2010). Evaluating the contribution of Interpretative Phenomenological Analysis. *Health Psychology Review.*

Smith, J.A., Flowers, P. & Larkin, M. (2009). *Interpretative phenomenological analysis: Theory, research, practice.* London: Sage.

Thompson, A.R., Smith, J.A. & Larkin, M. (in press). Interpretative phenomenological analysis and clinical psychology training: Results from a survey of the group of trainers in clinical psychology. *Clinical Psychology Forum.*

Further reading and useful website

Web

www.ipa.bbk.ac.uk. Home page for IPA with information on further reading, events and access to a discussion group.

Phenomenology

There is an introduction to the phenomenological background of IPA in Smith et al. (2009) but also see Langdridge (2007). For doctoral-level research, it can be advisable to engage with this material in more detail; Moran (2000) and then Dreyfus (2007) can be helpful resources.

IPA

Smith et al. (2009) provides more detailed exposition on most of the issues discussed here.

9

Existentialist-Informed Hermeneutic Phenomenology

Carla Willig and Abigail Billin

This chapter introduces a version of the phenomenological method that is particularly suitable for the exploration of embodied human experience. Like Interpretative Phenomenological Analysis (IPA), which was introduced in the preceding chapter, hermeneutic phenomenology belongs to the interpretative strand of phenomenology. This means that as a method of qualitative data analysis it seeks to capture and portray the quality and texture of research participants' experience and to explore its meanings and significance. In order to do this, hermeneutic phenomenology, like IPA, acknowledges the importance of the frames of reference which the researcher brings to the data during the process of analysis. Indeed, all forms of interpretative phenomenology take the view that interpretation is both desirable and inevitable; desirable because it serves to amplify the meanings contained in accounts of experience, and inevitable because understanding of an account cannot take place without us making some preliminary assumptions about its meaning. From this point of view, understanding involves a movement from presupposition to interpretation and back again, whereby the researcher's presuppositions (e.g., about the meaning of a word or the significance of an expression) are tested in the light of the evolving meaning of the account he or she is trying to understand and make sense of. This process has been referred to as the hermeneutic circle (for a helpful introduction to hermeneutics see Schmidt, 2006). It follows that in hermeneutic phenomenology the researcher both works with and continually challenges their own background knowledge, assumptions and presuppositions.

Qualitative Research Methods in Mental Health and Psychotherapy: A Guide for Students and Practitioners, First Edition. Edited by D. Harper and A.R. Thompson.
© 2012 John Wiley & Sons, Ltd. Published 2012 by John Wiley & Sons, Ltd.

Influences and Affinities

Hermeneutic phenomenology has affinities with existential philosophy. Van Manen (1990, p. 101) proposes that '[A]ll phenomenological human science research efforts are really explorations into the structure of the human lifeworld'. Although there are innumerable, and unique specific lifeworlds, corresponding to the wide range of possible and actual human realities and existences, there are also fundamental existential concerns which form part of the structure of the human lifeworld in general. These have been examined by existential philosophers such as (perhaps most famously) Martin Heidegger (e.g., Heidegger, 1962).

Fundamental existential themes include our relationship with time, our bodies, our physical environment and with other people. From an existential point of view, as humans we cannot but engage with these concerns in one way or another even if our way of engaging with them is characterized by a refusal to engage – think of the hermit whose way of engaging with the social is to exclude it from everyday life. Existentialist-informed hermeneutic phenomenological research involves both participant and researcher in a process of trying to make sense of what it means to 'be (human)', that is to say, what it means to live as an embodied being in a (particular) physical and social world. We want to emphasize that phenomenological exploration involves more than trying to understand what a participant is thinking. Whilst thoughts (i.e., a participant's ideas, beliefs, memories and so on in relation to a particular topic) are important, there is (much) more to human experience than this. Phenomenological exploration requires that the researcher engages with the participant's felt sense, their experience of 'how it is' for them to be in a particular situation, of 'what it is like' to have a particular experience. This is why existentialist-informed hermeneutic phenomenology is particularly suitable for the exploration of embodied human experience.

Epistemology

The aim of existentialist-informed hermeneutic phenomenological research is primarily to deepen our understanding of the quality, texture and meaning of a particular experience for those who undergo that experience. In addition, we may also seek to gain further insights into the human condition and to find out more about the many ways in which people can engage with fundamental existential concerns. Epistemologically this means that such research may be described as constructivist (Ponterotto, 2005) or contextual constructionist (Madill et al., 2000) in that the knowledge sought is knowledge about how participants are constructing meaning within particular contexts. Phenomenological knowledge is knowledge about the subjective experience of research participants. As such it can be contrasted with both realist knowledge (which seeks to identify the social and/or psychological processes or structures that underpin subjective experience) and social constructionist knowledge (which seeks to find out how people construct versions of social reality through the use of cultural resources such as discourses and symbolic practices).

Phenomenological knowledge aims to *understand* human experience. In order to do this, the researcher needs to find a way of getting as close as possible to the research participant's experience, to step into their shoes and to look at the world through their eyes – in other words, to enter their world. This means that the researcher assumes that there is more than one 'world' that can be studied. The question driving phenomenological research is, therefore, 'What is the world like *for this participant?*' (for a more detailed discussion of the epistemological bases of qualitative research including phenomenological research see Willig, in press).

Research Questions

Existentialist-informed hermeneutic phenomenology lends itself to the exploration of embodied human experiences which speak to our relationship with time, with our bodies, our physical environment and with other people. The kinds of research questions this method is best suited to address are concerned with lived experience and meaning-making. They are questions about what it may be like to undergo major life events, transitions between life stages, and physical or psychological transformations. They are questions about the ways in which we as humans negotiate and process fundamental existential concerns. Such research can focus directly on experiential phenomena (such as suffering, love, anger or joy) or it can attempt to access them through exploring participants' experiences of particular situations (such as being diagnosed with a medical condition, being made redundant, getting married or giving birth to a child). In either case, the focus of the research is upon the ways in which participants themselves interpret their experiences.

In addition, as indicated earlier, existentialist-informed hermeneutic phenomenology is interested in understanding participants' embodied experience, not simply in recording their thoughts and reflections about an experience. This means that such research needs to find ways of capturing and representing those aspects of experience that can be hard to talk about. For example, Radley (1993) draws attention to the importance of embodied practices (such as gardening) in the experience of recovering (a sense of being healthy) after major illness. Existentialist-informed hermeneutic phenomenological research is challenging in that it requires the researcher to engage with the (the meaning of) 'being' (human) as such rather than staying with participants' cognitions. Because of its holistic orientation, which foregrounds the unity of the mind–body complex, this approach to research has been embraced particularly by researchers in nursing studies (e.g., Cohen *et al.*, 2000; Lemon & Taylor, 1997). Langdridge (2007) identifies a number of examples of hermeneutic phenomenological research relevant to the area of mental health including a study on client experiences of psychotherapy (Sherwood, 2001), one on living with severe mental illness (Dalhberg *et al.*, 2001) and one on the meaning of parental bereavement (Lyndall *et al.*, 2005).

Existentialist-informed hermeneutic phenomenological research is ideally suited to address questions about what it is like to traverse existential challenges and how people make life meaningful and how they experience their world as a result. Along with most qualitative research, however, it is not suited to answer questions about relationships between variables or about cause–effect relationships. It is not designed to generate predictive models of behaviour nor does it allow us to generalize findings or to draw conclusions about the experiences of those who did not take part in the research. However, it does aim to generate insights into the nature of human experience which means that it is interested in particular individuals' subjective experiences only in so far as they shed light on the phenomenon of interest. In other words, existentialist-informed phenomenological research is primarily concerned with experiential phenomena (e.g., the phenomenon of suffering, of loss, of joy, etc.) rather than with the individuals whose accounts help the researcher to illuminate the phenomenon. Whilst its focus on individual subjective experience means that this type of research may appear to fail to provide us with much information about the wider social, cultural and historical contexts within which such experiences are located, it could be argued that in order to fully understand the meanings participants create and to fully appreciate their significance, the phenomenological researcher would need to locate them within their wider contexts (see also Chapter 8; Langdridge, 2007). This argument chimes with Gadamer's (1989) view that hermeneutics involves the study of texts in their widest sense (i.e., as tissues of meaning and signification) and that 'meaning takes place when a particular tradition – that is, the language of a group of people – is interpreted by a speaker' (Cohen et al., 2000, pp. 5–6). In other words, meaning is not created out of nothing, it is not conjured by individuals from meaninglessness; rather, meaning is made out of cultural resources (including language) whose availability depends upon socio-historical conditions. Thus, as Cohen et al. (2000, p. 6) conclude, 'the individual and the tradition must both be considered in hermeneutic phenomenology'.

Research Process

Phenomenological research is interested in (the quality, texture and meaning of) lived experience. Since it is impossible to directly access someone else's lived experience, phenomenological researchers rely upon descriptive accounts of experience. Such accounts can be spoken or written, and they can be supported by the use of images or music and sounds. Data for phenomenological research can take the form of recordings and transcriptions of semi-structured interviews, of written or spoken recollections of experiences, video-diaries produced by research participants or, indeed, of other types of visual data (see Reavey, 2011). Whatever form the data take, it is important to remember that such accounts are already one step removed from the original lived experience itself; therefore, they constitute transformations of the experience (see van Manen, 1990, p. 54). Furthermore, it is easy for phenomenological research to further transform the data in such a way as to lose the original account's emotional tone and vibrancy. This happens when the researcher analyses the account by extracting and labelling themes, which capture the content but not the felt sense of what has been described (for a discussion of this process see Willig, 2007). Van Manen (1997) has argued that the thematic dimension in phenomenological inquiry tends to dominate the expressive dimension, and that it is important that we find ways of letting the emotional tone of our research participants' narratives speak to the readers of our research texts. Ohlen (2003, p. 565) endorses van Manen's (1997) critique when he observes that the formal and rational language used by researchers 'does not have the power to give life to the mysteries of life'. In order to redress the balance, these researchers recommend the use of poetic narrative in the analysis of accounts. These are constructed from direct quotations from research participants, with the aim of evoking the original experience. According to van Manen (1997, p. 353), '[E]vocation means that experience is brought vividly into presence so that we can phenomenologically reflect on it.'

Phenomenological analysis is a very time-consuming and demanding process. This means that researchers tend to work with relatively small numbers of participants in any one study. Because the aim of the analysis is to shed light on the nature and essence of a particular human experience, participants need to be recruited on the basis of their ability to provide accounts that will illuminate the quality, texture and meaning of that experience. This means that they need to have had the experience and they need to be able and willing to reflect on it in some detail and in some depth. The quality of a phenomenological analysis depends to a large extent on the richness of the data. It is difficult, if not impossible, to produce a fertile reading of a very short, monosyllabic account (although, of course, the very absence of colour and texture from an account may tell us something rather important about the quality of the experience). It follows that the applicability of the phenomenological method is limited by its dependence upon 'high quality' accounts and the consequent exclusion of the experiences of those who may not be able to articulate them in the (relatively) sophisticated manner required by the method (see also Willig, 2008, pp. 67–68).

Role of Research Participants

Because phenomenological research aims to capture the quality, texture and meaning of research participants' experiences, one might expect that one way of validating one's findings would be to check with participants that one 'has got it right'. This is indeed advocated by some phenomenological researchers (e.g., Colaizzi, 1978; Cohen *et al.*, 2000). Indeed, research participants in phenomenological research are often referred to as 'co-researchers' in order to emphasize their active participation in what can be a highly collaborative research process. For example, Colaizzi (1978) recommends that, following data analysis, the researcher returns to the participants with a descriptive account of the phenomenon under investigation in order to find out to what extent the researcher's account reflects their original experiences. Each participant is invited to let the researcher know whether any important aspects of their experience have been omitted from the account and whether the account contains anything that does not fit with their original experience. Participants' comments are then used to produce a revised version of the account. The process of validation continues, by taking the revised account back to the participants for further validation. This cycle of validation contin-ues until there are no more revisions to the researcher's account. However, Colaizzi's

(1978) approach to phenomenological research is descriptive rather than interpretative, which means that participant validation of the findings is a much more straight-forward process than it is for more interpretative approaches such as hermeneutic phenomenology. Langdridge (2007, pp. 81–82) identifies three challenges associated with seeking participants' feedback on the analysis. First, there is the issue of accessibility of the analysis. Langdridge (2007) points out that in order to obtain meaningful feedback, the researcher would need to ensure that the analysis is written in accessible language and that it is explained to participants if necessary. This, although desirable, is not always practically possible. Secondly, there is the issue of power. Participants may find it difficult to provide feedback which they feel may be interpreted as a challenge to or a criticism of the researcher's analysis. Finally, Langdridge (2007) argues that because an interpretative approach to phenomenology takes the analysis beyond the original description provided by the participant, it is possible that participants may not recognize the interpretation as being relevant to their experience. This does not necessarily mean that the researcher has 'got it wrong'. It may be that the participant retains a partial perspective on their experience, perhaps in order to avoid confronting some (perhaps painful or disturbing) aspects of their experience. In this case, there are also ethical concerns about a research process that brings participants face-to-face with potential meanings of their experience which they may not be ready or willing to engage with. After all, agreeing to take part in a research project is not the same as entering a therapeutic relationship.

An Example of Existentialist-Informed Hermeneutic Phenomenology

To demonstrate how to use existentialist-informed hermeneutic phenomenology, we describe a study conducted in order to explore the process of meaning-making at the end of life (for a more detailed account of this research see Taylor, 2009). Finding meaning when facing a diagnosis of advanced cancer can be a challenging experience as it requires engagement with some of the dimensions of human existence (such as mortality and suffering) which may not be foregrounded when we are healthy and feeling well. Spirituality has frequently been cited as an important source of meaning, yet there is no consensus over what this term actually means. We were interested in exploring how those who are facing the lived reality of their own mortality make sense of this experience. We wanted to know more about how meaning is made of life when its end is in sight. We were also interested in the extent to which 'spirituality' is a meaningful concept within this context.

Aims of the study

Given that spirituality is such a difficult concept to define, we started the research with an open, orientating question: what is the experience of 'spirituality' and meaning-making at the end of life? The word 'spirituality' was left undefined to allow participants to explore their own definitions during the research. In order to allow participants to decide for themselves whether or not 'spirituality' was relevant to their experience, we made it clear in our recruitment materials that we were primarily interested in their experience of the end of life and that 'spirituality' may or may not be a part of this.

A hermeneutic phenomenological method was employed because this was considered a creative approach to explore such an elusive concept. Van Manen's (1990) hermeneutic phenomenological technique was chosen as it offered the openness and flexibility required by our research question. Van Manen (1990) emphasizes that there is no prescribed method in hermeneutic phenomenology. Instead, he argues that the focus of phenomenology should always be on creative engagement with language in order to reveal something that was previously concealed.

Data collection

Eight participants (three males and five females) were recruited from a hospice, with ages ranging from 44 to 80 years. Participants identified themselves as wanting to talk about their experience of 'spirituality' and meaning-making and as being in the advanced stages of cancer, defined as having a life expectancy of less than 1 year. Because the concept of 'spirituality' was left undefined in the research question, there was a risk that individuals would not consider themselves appropriate for the study depending on their definition of 'spirituality'. To avoid excluding potential participants, it was explained to potential participants that 'spirituality' did not necessarily have to imply religion and was only a suggested label to describe their experience of finding meaning in their experience.

Data were collected in the form of relatively unstructured interviews conducted by the second author. This is a popular method when using hermeneutic phenomenology because it helps the researcher to take a fresh look at the phenomenon without imposing any preconceived ideas (van Manen, 1990). Also the pace and timing of this kind of interview is flexible and can be adjusted to the individual, which was particularly important given that participants may have had limited concentration spans as a result of pain or fatigue.

Participants were told that we wanted to understand their experience of 'spirituality', or whatever term they preferred to use, and how they made sense of life at the end of life. The opening question in the interviews ('What is life like for you at the moment?') was broad and open-ended. Further clarifying and probing questions were then asked to facilitate rich descriptions of participants' experiences.

Given that understanding in hermeneutic phenomenology is a product of reflections on interpretations and experience, a reflexive diary was kept by the second author throughout the research to record thoughts and feelings during the study. An important aspect of interpretative phenomenology is inter-subjectivity, particularly with respect to how the researcher influences the research process. Keeping a reflexive diary ensured that the researcher was not separated from the findings. For example, when she felt surprised about the results she considered what this told her about her own preconceptions.

Similarly, she considered how her own good health might have shaped the way people spoke to her, and what message they might have been trying to give to someone who is not close to death.

Analysis

The purpose of a phenomenological inquiry is to make us 'see' something in a manner that enriches our understanding of experience, not just cognitively but also emotionally. Ohlen (2003) proposed poetic condensation as a method that can engage the reader at a deeper level of meaning by preserving the expressive content of a narrative. The transcripts were therefore formulated into lines of poetry using Gee's (1991) model of poetic condensation by making use of accentuation, pauses and rhythm in the participant's speech. This meant that the interview transcripts were transformed into poems which then constituted the data to be analysed.

Hermeneutic phenomenology deliberately moves away from the mechanical application of coding to allow the researcher to engage in the 'free acting of "seeing"' (van Manen, 1990, p. 79). Van Manen (1990) suggests three approaches to analysing data whilst engaging in the hermeneutic circle of moving between the parts and the whole of the data in the process of distilling meaning:

1. *Holistic reading.* This involves attending to the text as a whole and finding phrases that capture the fundamental meaning of the text as a whole.
2. *Selective reading.* This requires reading the text several times to find sentences or phrases that seem particularly significant, essential or revealing.
3. *Detailed reading.* This is achieved by reading every single sentence or sentence cluster and analysing what the sentence reveals about the phenomenon.

The analysis was supplemented by the reflexive observations noted during data collection and the analytic process. As each poem was analysed, the previous poems were used to help enhance the analytic process, rather than as a source of comparison. Thus, another dialogue between the parts and the whole was established by thinking about one poem in the context of all the poems, as well as comparing the parts and the whole within the text. This shifting back and forth between the parts and the whole revealed new issues and new questions which were then used to further interrogate the data.

For van Manen (1990), writing is not a process that characterizes the final stage of research, but instead is an essential part of the hermeneutic phenomenological investigation. Consequently, the analysis involved a constant writing and rewriting of reflections on the parts and the whole, showing a clear trail of evolving thought. Each analysis of individual participants' interviews as well as the reflections on the overall experience was written and rewritten several times. Themes were derived as a way of creating structure and making sense of the phenomenon rather than the result of a formal application of coding. The process of generating themes in hermeneutic phenomenology is less prescriptive than in most other qualitative approaches as it is derived from the researcher's dialogue with the text (van Manen, 1990).

Findings

Analysis revealed two modes of being that were available to the participants: the *everyday mode of being* and the *transcendent mode of being.* These had implications for the experience of 'spirituality' and meaning-making at the end of life. The modes of being were not mutually exclusive and there were times when participants would change their mode of being depending on the context of their environment.

For participants in the everyday mode of being, the experience of 'spirituality' and meaning-making was associated with doing their usual everyday activities. By carrying on with their everyday lives despite their physical limitations, individuals in the everyday mode of being felt a sense of belonging in the physical world and being physically present with other human beings. For example, in the following extract Sandra emphasizes the importance of making an effort in order to ensure that she was able to share memorable and joyful experiences with her children whilst this was still possible:

> I try and do things with the kids
> My son's 16 and we went to the zoo on Thursday because he was on half-term
> And we had such a fantastic time
>
> It was really nice
> On his sixteenth birthday
> It cost me an arm and a leg
> But I hired him a mini bus, took all his friends to paintballing
> So things that they can all remember together (Sandra[1])

Having a relationship with another human being was an important source of meaning in the everyday mode of being. The quality of these relationships was fundamental, because participants expressed the need to have people connect with them as a person and not a patient. By interacting with their family, friends or the hospice (as referred to in the next quote) they retained their sense of belongingness to the social world, reducing their sense of isolation.

> Coming here helps because you meet other people
> You know that are suffering just like you.
> And you see some of them that are worse
> Often than myself
>
> And when you meet with other people who have it as well
> You can talk
> And they can tell you how they feel
> And you can say how you feel (Lucas)

---

[1] All names have been changed to protect anonymity.

The participants in the everyday mode of being did not want to spend time on their own reflecting on their situation. Their experience of 'spirituality' and meaning-making was associated with gathering their inner resources to carry on with life. They felt that they wanted and needed to be strong to face the physical demands of their existence and carry on with their physical interactions and social relationships.

> And even now
> Even though the doctors have said
> Well the Macmillan nurse said that it might have been my last Christmas
> I feel strong enough, I reckon I can see the next Christmas (Sandra)

'Spirituality' and meaning-making in the everyday mode of being was associated with a strong sense of purpose and future goals. It was about letting the world and other people matter, to remain invested and interested in the social world and to maintain a connection with it. The awareness of temporal limits made life's purpose more pressured, and idle time was seen as wasted time. In this mode, participants also thought a lot about their local community and were concerned about how people's behaviour and social policies affected their immediate world.

> There was a program on TV last night
> I think somewhere in north London
> One big estate will be without electricity and gas, water for the rest of the year right over Christmas
> And yet they send all this money overseas
> Instead of getting this country organized properly.
>
> I mean I believe in charities to a certain extent
> But the truth is
> That charity always begins at home (Bob)

For those in the transcendent mode of being, interacting with their day-to-day physical and social world as specific individuals was not as meaningful as for those in the everyday mode of being. Instead, viewing themselves as part of a whole and understanding how they fit into the bigger picture was important to their experience of 'spirituality' and helped them create meaning. In this mode of being, participants did not focus on their individual physical bodies. Instead, they meditated on the pattern of the universe and thought about how their lives were only a tiny part of a much bigger whole.

> I went to a place right in the South of Japan
> And there is a volcano there
> It was actually billowing
> It was sort of more or less alive
>
> And the whole earth
> Trembled
> It was just an amazing thing
> The power of it was just immense
> And you realize what an insignificant little bunch we are. (John)

Participants' experience of 'spirituality' and meaning-making in the transcendent mode of being involved detaching from unhelpful relationships in order to maintain their peace and quiet. Connecting with people at the hospice and those who understood their perspective was still key to their experience but these relationships were few and far between. They found meaning from their relationships with their family, but there was a need to not over-attach in order to prepare them for their death.

> I need to not become involved
> Just stay happy in the other world, in my world where I want to be
> I feel that I can let go
> There's nothing stopping me
> Not people demanding (Kate)

In the transcendent mode of being, participants identified reflecting on their being-in-the-world as a fundamental part of their experience of 'spirituality' and meaning-making. Their sense of self became more fluid as they detached from their physical and social worlds, transcending their immediate reality and reviewing what mattered to them now that they were dying.

> What is life like at the moment?
> Peaceful and quiet
> Well I attempt to make it as peaceful and quiet
> And withdrawing really from the well world
>
> I sort of divide into the well world and the ill world
> Where I am
> And I don't want to be in the well world
> There are just so many demands I am not really interested in anymore
>
> I want to be in this side (Kate)

In the transcendent mode of being, an important part of the experience of 'spirituality' was finding meaning from thinking about the whole of the world or universe. Participants felt that they had fulfilled their purpose and had nothing left to do. They were living in the present moment and not driven towards a goal in the future other than death itself. Having individual beliefs was important for their experience of 'spirituality' and meaning-making, in terms of politics and religion. It seemed as though their thoughts about the state of the world reflected their reduced need for individual meaning and instead increased their desire to think about collective meaning.

> What is my purpose in life?
> That has gone now
> Because I have lived my life
> I have raised my three children
>
> I thought that I'll probably sat down and talk with them and say I have no regrets
> Maybe I might have done some of it differently
> I have no regrets
> I enjoy my life (Edith)

Conclusions

Our existentialist-informed hermeneutic phenomenological analysis of the data has identified different ways of making sense of life when living with advanced cancer. Finding meaning in life at the end of life can take the form of maintaining a connection with the social world (via the everyday mode of being) or it can take the form of detaching from the physical and social world and one's personal investment in it (via the transcendent mode). The transcendent mode of being offered meaning by transcending the personal, individual situation of being terminally ill and viewing the world from afar. In contrast, the everyday mode of being offered meaning through the experience of belonging-in-the-world. These two modes of being have important implications for the way the person experiences the givens of existence (van Manen, 1990). In the everyday mode of being, primary meaning is found in lived human relations and the enhancement of positive relationships in one's life. In contrast, in the transcendent mode of being, withdrawal from lived human relations and a turning towards one's inner self become more meaningful. It was interesting to note that the decision to stop treatment seemed to be associated with the transcendent mode of being. However, it is important to stress that people can, and do, move between the two modes, depending on the context within which they find themselves. Regarding the usefulness of the notion of 'spirituality', although some of our participants (particularly when in the transcendent mode of being) did use the term, we conclude that what mattered to participants was that their lives remained meaningful and valuable and that 'spirituality' seems to be very much in the eye of the beholder.

Reflections

We hope that our example of an existentialist-informed hermeneutic phenomenological study has demonstrated how this method can be used in order to distil, capture and foreground meanings which structure the human experience of the end of life. We want to conclude by offering some reflections on how one may go about evaluating this type of research and how it might be used in order to inform practice. As one of us has argued elsewhere (Willig, in press) whilst the criteria traditionally used to evaluate quantitative research (i.e., reliability, representativeness, generalizability, objectivity and validity) are not applicable to qualitative research, such research does involve a process of systematic, cyclical, critical reflection whose quality can be assessed. However, the criteria we use for evaluating a qualitative study must be informed by the study's epistemological position. In the case of existentialist-informed hermeneutic phenomenology, this means that scrutiny of the study's use of reflexivity and the researcher's awareness of their use of their own thoughts and feelings about what the participant is saying in order to uncover meaning will be an important part of an evaluation. In addition, an examination of the extent to which the study explores (and ideally theorizes) the relationship between accounts (i.e., both the participants' accounts, that is to say the data, as well as the researcher's analytic account) and the context(s) within which these have been produced, would also be useful. Regarding the usefulness of this type of research we would argue that an increased awareness of the diverse ways in which people engage with fundamental existential concerns and how this can be shaped by the (social, psychological, material) contexts within which they find themselves, can only improve social–psychological policy formulations and interventions.

References

Cohen, M.Z., Kahn, D. & Steeves, R.H. (2000). *Hermeneutic phenomenological research: A practical guide for nurse researchers*. London: Sage.

Colaizzi, P. (1978). Psychological research as the phenomenologist views it. In R. Valle & M. King (Eds.) *Existential-phenomenological alternatives for psychology*. New York: Oxford University Press.

Dahlberg, K., Drew, N. & Nystrom, M. (2001). *Reflective lifeworld research*. Lund, Sweden: Studentlitteratur.

Gadamer, H.G. (1989). *Truth and method* (2nd edn.; Trans. J. Weinsheimer & D.G. Marshall). New York: Crossroads.

Gee, J.P. (1991). A linguistic approach to narrative. *Journal of Narrative and Life History, 1* (1), 15–39.

Heidegger, M. (1962). Being and time (Trans. J. Macquarrie & E. Robinson). Oxford: Basil Blackwell.

Langdridge, D. (2007). *Phenomenological psychology: Theory, research and method*. Harlow: Pearson.

Lemon, N. & Taylor, H. (1997). Caring in casualty: The phenomenology of nursing care. In N. Hayes (Ed.) *Doing qualitative analysis in psychology* (pp. 227–244). Hove: Psychology Press.

Lyndall, A.M., Pretorius, G. & Stuart, A. (2005). Give sorrow words: The meaning of parental bereavement. *Indio-Pacific Journal of Phenomenology, 5* (2), 1–12.

Madill, A., Jordan, A. & Shirley, C. (2000). Objectivity and reliability in qualitative analysis: Realist, contextualist and radical constructionist epistemologies. *British Journal of Psychology, 91*, 1–20.

Ohlen, J. (2003). Evocation of meaning through poetic condensation of narratives in empirical phenomenological inquiry into human suffering. *Qualitative Health Research, 13*, 557–566.

Ponterotto, J.G. (2005). Qualitative research in counseling psychology: A primer on research paradigms and philosophy of science. *Journal of Counseling Psychology, 52* (2), 126–136.

Radley, A. (1993). The role of metaphor in adjustment to chronic illness. In A. Radley (Ed.) *Worlds of illness: Biographical and cultural perspectives on health and disease* (pp. 109–123). London: Routledge.

Reavey, P. (Ed.) (2011). *Visual psychologies: Using and interpreting images in qualitative research*. London: Psychology Press.

Schmidt, L.K. (2006). *Understanding hermeneutics*. Stocksfield: Acumen.

Sherwood, T. (2001). Client experience in psychotherapy: What heals and what harms? *Indio-Pacific Journal of Phenomenology, 1* (2), 1–16.

Taylor, A. (2009). Dying-in-the-world: An exploration of 'spirituality' and meaning-making at the end of life. *DPsych portfolio on integrating the mind and the body: Examining the role of counselling psychology for individuals with physical health problems*. City University, London.

van Manen, M. (1990). *Researching the lived experience: Human science for an action sensitive pedagogy.* Ontario: Althouse Press.

van Manen, M. (1997). *Researching the lived experience: Human science for an action sensitive pedagogy* (2nd edn.) Ontario: Althouse Press.

Willig, C. (2007). Reflections on the use of the phenomenological method. *Qualitative Research in Psychology, 4,* 1–17.

Willig, C. (2008). *Introducing qualitative research in psychology* (2nd edn). Maidenhead: McGraw Hill/Open University Press.

Willig, C. (in press). Perspectives on the epistemological bases of qualitative research. In H. Cooper (Ed.) *The handbook of research methods in psychology.* Washington: American Psychological Association Books.

Further Reading

Cohen, M.Z., Kahn, D. & Steeves, R.H. (2000). *Hermeneutic phenomenological research: A practical guide for nurse researchers.* London: Sage.

Cohn, H.W. (2005). Interpretation: Explanation or understanding? In E. van Duerzen & C. Arnold-Baker (Eds.) *Existential perspectives on human issues: A handbook for therapeutic practice.* Basingstoke: Palgrave Macmillan.

Jacobson, B. (2007). *Invitation to existential psychology.* Chichester: Wiley.

Langdridge, D. (2007). *Phenomenological psychology: Theory, research and method.* London: Pearson Prentice Hall.

van Manen, M. (1997). *Researching the lived experience: Human science for an action sensitive pedagogy* (2nd edn). Ontario: Althouse Press.

10

Grounded Theory Methods for Mental Health Practitioners

Alison Tweed and Kathy Charmaz

History of Grounded Theory

Grounded theory as a qualitative methodology was developed by Barney G. Glaser and Anselm L. Strauss, two sociologists investigating the social processes of death and dying in hospital in the United States in the mid 1960s. Their book, *The Discovery of Grounded Theory* (Glaser & Strauss, 1967), explicated a rigorous set of inductively driven research strategies, designed to proceed systematically from a set of specific observations to a general conclusion or theory in order to describe and conceptualize people's views, actions and life experiences within the context in which they are lived. Their methods contrasted to dominant positivistic and quantitative forms of research at that time. Positivistic forms of research focused on experimentation and observation to empirically test and verify hypotheses as a means of describing the world in measurable variables. Glaser and Strauss highlighted qualitative methods of inquiry as a legitimate form of research in their own right. Grounded theory gained popularity in certain disciplines such as nursing over the next decade and was used in 1970s mental health research. Wilson's (1977) major mental health nursing study in the United States analysed over 200 hours of observation and interview data from a community setting for people diagnosed with schizophrenia. However, grounded theory did not begin to gain favour within psychology until another decade later. Psychologists initially conceptualized it for use within clinical and health psychology as a fruitful means of gaining alternative and in-depth perspectives of service users' experiences (e.g., Rennie *et al.*, 1988).

Glaser and Strauss each brought a unique set of assumptions to the development of grounded theory as a method: Glaser brought positivist notions of objectivity based upon his quantitative background whereas Strauss took a pragmatist stance, influenced by an interest in action, language and meaning. Whilst these epistemological differences

Qualitative Research Methods in Mental Health and Psychotherapy: A Guide for Students and Practitioners, First Edition.
Edited by D. Harper and A.R. Thompson.
© 2012 John Wiley & Sons, Ltd. Published 2012 by John Wiley & Sons, Ltd.

could be argued as adding multiple dimensions to the method, they eventually led to Glaser and Strauss's alternative forms of grounded theory. Today, scholars view grounded theory's epistemological position as operating on a continuum from more positivist forms (Glaser, 1992) through post-positivist (Strauss & Corbin, 1990) to constructivist versions[1] (Charmaz, 2006; for a review see Madill *et al.*, 2000).

Introduction to the Method

The grounded theory method provides explicit strategies for data collection and analysis and aims to produce an inductively driven theory of social or psychological processes *grounded* in the material from which it was derived. Most typically, textual material has been the primary form of data, including interview transcripts, written documents and diaries. Glaser and Strauss (1967) outlined a number of characteristics of grounded theory, including the simultaneous involvement in collecting and analysing data, the development of analytic codes and categories and making comparisons between codes, concepts and categories.

Starting with the data itself, developing a grounded theory can be conceptualized as a *pyramid*, where the raw data and the basic descriptive codes ascribed to the meaning-units of this data form the building blocks; the foundational base of the pyramid as it were. Focused codes and categories form the additional, less numerous blocks of the pyramid. These codes and categories conceptualize the basic codes beneath them and the pyramid builds towards its peak, each level denoting a higher, more sophisticated level of abstraction and interpretation. Finally comes the peak of the pyramid either representing a core category, encompassing all those codes and categories subsumed within it; or a theoretical conceptualization of the processes interpreted from the data. Here is the pinnacle of the analysis from which the storyline of the grounded theory can be conveyed to others.

In addition to the principles outlined above, grounded theorists also use a series of analytical and reflexive strategies to aid the process of developing theory. The first of these is the constant comparative method (Glaser & Strauss, 1967). Here, all elements of the analysis – data, codes, categories and concepts – are constantly compared within and between each other. This comparative process entails looking for similarities, differences and nuances between all the elements of the analysis in order to generate a more abstract understanding of the material. Using this comparative method is a dynamic non-linear process, requiring the researcher to stay open to new insights within the analysis.

Assisting this process is the second strategy of memo-writing (Charmaz, 2006). Memo-writing is an intermediate stage between data collection and write-up and involves the detailed capturing of the researcher's thoughts, hunches, interpretations and decision-making throughout the analysis. We can view memo-writing as part of the

---

[1] Whilst there is an accepted difference between constructivist and social constructionist perspectives within the United Kingdom, the term 'constructivist grounded theory' has become widely used in the both the UK and US research literatures. The worked example and approach presented in this chapter is consistent with a contemporary UK social constructionist approach.

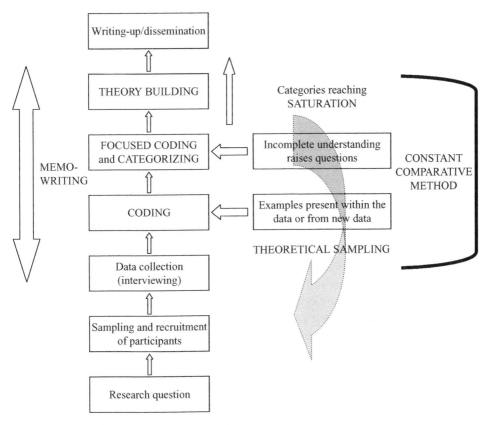

Figure 10.1   Visual representation of a grounded theory.

'audit trail' of grounded theory, enabling the recording of the analysis as it happens. We provide detailed examples of coding and memo-writing below to show how grounded theorists use these strategies.

Finally, theoretical sampling is a strategy designed to sample new cases or data actively in order to develop, refine and elaborate the emerging grounded theory. Researchers engage in theoretical sampling *after* they have developed tentative analytic categories. Thus, theoretical sampling is unrelated to purposive sampling or representative sampling conducted at the beginning of the research process. Memos can alert the researcher to under-developed areas of theory, gaps or hypotheses requiring elaboration or testing. Here, the purely inductive emphasis of grounded theory alters because theoretical sampling contains both inductive and deductive elements. Typical theoretical sampling questions might be: 'Whose voices are not represented by my tentative category?' or 'Who do I need to speak to next to develop this theoretical category?' Ideally, theoretical sampling of new material continues until saturation is reached. Here, no new insights or development of the theory or properties of categories occur through the gathering of additional data. Depending on the scope of the research question, with interview transcripts saturation may occur after collecting considerable data or after checking key analytic categories through theoretical sampling of selected interviewees who possess the requisite knowledge to shed light on the properties of these categories (Charmaz, 2006).

In order to aid the reader, Figure 10.1 presents a visual representation of the process of developing a grounded theory. The example uses interview transcripts as data and illustrates all the key elements from data gathering to dissemination.

What Kinds of Research Questions is Grounded Theory Most Suited To?

Grounded theory's theoretical, epistemological and technical foundations position it well to investigate a broad range of open-ended research questions that focus on processes, patterns and meaning within context and that require the crucial examination of subjectivity of experience and thus lead researchers to begin inquiry from their research participants' point of view. Grounded theory can be employed where existing theories or areas of research are under-defined or patchy and has the flexibility and sensitivity to be responsive to changing contexts and conditions (Henwood & Pidgeon, 2003). In other words, grounded theory methods foster specifying the implications of changes in social settings and situations where the studied phenomenon occurs as well as delineating the conditions under which it arises, is maintained, or varies. It is not surprising therefore that grounded theory has gained popularity as a method within mental health research and it has frequently been used to analyse the accounts of those individuals and groups typically perceived as 'marginalized' (see, e.g., Boyd & Gumley, 2007; Charmaz, 2008; Charmaz & Rosenfeld, 2006; Karp, 1996). Further, a review of recently published grounded theory articles provides additional examples: clients' experiences of disengaged moments in psychotherapy (Frankel & Levitt, 2009), transition to motherhood for women with postnatal depression (Homewood *et al.*, 2009), perceptions of the concept of recovery from schizophrenia (Noiseux & Ricard, 2008) and nurses' experiences of working in acute psychiatric settings (Chiovitti, 2008).

However, grounded theory is not solely focused on individuals' interpretation of their experience but has a broader remit. Primarily, the goal of grounded theory is to develop an inductively driven theory of studying basic social or psychological processes (Glaser & Strauss, 1967) in which the researcher defines a fundamental process occurring in the setting or among the research participants and pursues researching it as the phenomenon of interest. The focus on social processes enables grounded theory to investigate how social structures, situations and relationships influence patterns of behaviour, interactions and interpretations. This focus can include the impact of policies and services upon behaviour (e.g., Wuest *et al.*, 2006). With apparent parallels in terms of researcher reflexivity and the self-reflection of therapists, psychotherapists have also seen grounded theory as a suitable method for psychotherapy research including systemic therapy (Burck, 2005) and psychoanalytic research (Anderson, 2006).

What Kinds of Questions is Grounded Theory Not Suited To?

Madill and Gough (2008) have provided a useful positioning framework, outlining where grounded theory as an analytic method can be placed in relation to the variety of qualitative approaches available. Within this framework, Madill and Gough highlight four areas in which qualitative methods can be organized in terms of their procedural categorization: *discursive, thematic, structured* and *instrumental.* Grounded theory has been described as *thematic,* alongside other methods such as Interpretative Phenomenological Analysis (Smith, 1996) and Thematic Analysis (Braun & Clarke, 2006). Following this argument, grounded theory would not be suitable for 'testing out' existing theory or hypotheses, perhaps through the use of a priori domains or pre-designed coding schemes (*structural* methods). From a constructivist approach, neither is grounded theory a particularly suitable method for making truth statements or knowledge claims about an objective reality (Suddaby, 2006).

Collecting Data: What Constitutes Data and How Much Should I Collect?

Most commonly, grounded theory studies have been associated with the analysis of transcripts of interview data, typically gathered in a semi-structured format. However, this focus neglects the wide range of information that can be used as data and can provide novice researchers with a narrowed conceptualization of what constitutes data suitable for grounded theory analysis. Grounded theorists have used a number of sources of data including official records, letters and diary entries, fieldnotes based on observational work and focus group material, in addition to interview transcripts (for a summary see Henwood & Pidgeon, 2003). How each researcher views and works with data depends on his or her epistemological position. From a post-positivist frame, the data will be seen factually as a representation of reality; from a constructivist frame, the data will have been constructed for a specific purpose and outcome and needs to be recognized as such (Charmaz, 2006).

The amount of data to collect within a grounded theory study very much depends upon the research goal. Studies that are aiming to theorize will require greater amounts of data than those studies aiming to provide detailed descriptions of localized phenomena. Whilst pragmatic factors often play a part in determining the amount of data collected, it is the principle of saturation that should be the key consideration. Data collection ceases when theoretical categories are saturated (see previous section). In principle it sounds a relatively straightforward matter to determine whether categories are saturated, yet in actuality it is a complicated and challenging process and whilst it is easy to claim saturation, it is much more difficult to demonstrate it (Morse, 1995). Bowen (2008) argues that published grounded theory studies need to demonstrate the saturation process explicitly by providing clear descriptions and criteria used in the write-up. He provides an example of how this was achieved in his grounded theory investigation of community-based anti-poverty projects.

How Might Participants and Service Users be Involved in Grounded Theory Studies?

Undoubtedly, the most traditionally frequent form of participant involvement in a grounded theory study occurs during the data collection stage of the research. Here, the researcher actively seeks those individuals he or she believes can reveal something in relation to the phenomenon of interest. Yet to focus solely on the participant as the subjective focus of the research question as a means of eliciting data neglects those other areas where participants can successfully play a part. Charmaz (2006) discusses the notion of *sensitizing concepts*, a term originally described by Blumer (1969). Sensitizing concepts are seen as a starting point to grounded theory research through which the researcher generates initial ideas of interest, pays attention to guiding theoretical frameworks and becomes sensitized to asking particular types of questions, such as questions about identity or stigma. Participant involvement at this early stage can therefore be valuable in priming the researcher to key experiences of interest and providing a particular focus for the research. In an example of this, Boyd and Gumley (2007) undertook a grounded theory study with service users who had experiences of persecutory paranoia in order to develop an experiential perspective of this phenomenon. The authors were sensitized to the study by consultation with service users at the design stage who assisted in guiding the authors to particular areas of concern and relevance.

However, only a small minority of grounded theory studies have demonstrated a broader range of service user involvement. One example is the study undertaken by Rose *et al.* (2004) investigating consumers' views of electroconvulsive therapy (ECT) through the use of a variety of data sources. Two of the authors had been recipients of ECT themselves and whilst the paper does not fully discuss the influence of these experiences upon the research process, they clearly sensitized the researchers and could well have improved both their understanding and engagement with the gathered data. Teram *et al.* (2005) also used grounded theory (alongside participatory action research) in a study investigating female survivors of child sexual abuse and their experiences of physical therapy. They aimed to empower the research participants as a means of informing professional practice and training.

How Does a Researcher Use Grounded Theory?

What is coding?

Coding is the first step of the analytic process and involves taking data apart. When coding, researchers break their data into analysable fragments and name these fragments. Thus, a code is a shorthand analytic label that a researcher defines. Grounded theorists aim to make their codes active, short, specific and spontaneous (Charmaz, 2006).

Through coding, researchers gain an analytic handle on their material and an analytic point(s) of departure. Grounded theorists grapple with data and define their meanings through using codes. Coding serves the following objectives:

1. To engage researchers with their data without applying preconceived concepts;
2. To define what is happening in these data;
3. To compare, sort and categorize fragments of data; and
4. To begin connecting data with data, data with codes, and codes with codes.

Constructivist grounded theorists acknowledge how researchers' and their research participants' social locations and perspectives and the situation of inquiry shape data (see also Clarke, 2005). Thus, researchers should account for their starting points and standpoints and analyse how they affect inquiry. Keeping codes active and specific helps the researcher accomplish this objective.

Much research done in the name of grounded theory is descriptive and thematic. Thus, such research addresses topics as given rather than taking them apart and defining how they are constituted. Glaser and Strauss's (Glaser, 1978, 1998; Glaser & Strauss, 1967) early methodological strategies have always held potential for developing theoretical analyses. The grounded theory emphasis on analysing processes begins with using gerunds for coding. Because a gerund is the noun form of a verb, it preserves action by stating what people are doing, such as 'defining', 'explaining' or 'accounting'. Gerunds also facilitate making connections between data and between codes. Thus, the researcher gains a handle on a greater portion of the data and links actions and events to reveal the story in the data, to invoke Strauss's focus.[2] Coding with gerunds enables psychologists to:

1. Study emergent phenomena comparatively;
2. Make implicit meanings, actions and processes more visible and tangible;
3. Define relationships between inner mental processes and external events;
4. Provide initial but modifiable conceptual handles for understanding and sorting large amounts of data; and
5. Construct successively more abstract theoretical categories and relationships.

Inductive coding data has permeated qualitative research, although coding with gerunds has not. Most researchers code for topics and themes at a considerably more general level than actions represented by gerunds. Topics or themes aid in sorting and synthesizing data but seldom break them apart as readily or make implicit relationships as visible as does coding for actions with gerunds (Charmaz, in press). Topics and themes tend to separate data into discrete units rather than reveal links between them.

In addition to coding with gerunds, grounded theorists code small units of data. Line-by-line coding with gerunds is a heuristic device to bring the researcher into the data, interact with it and study each fragment of it (Box 10. 1). Line-by-line coding means giving each line in the data a short label to capture what the researcher defines is happening in each datum. Line-by-line coding is particularly helpful for analysing in-depth interviews or personal accounts. Using this type of coding during initial data collection assists researchers in defining directions to explore, helps them identify gaps in their data and spurs them to compare data and codes. Line-by-line coding with gerunds generates leads to pursue in subsequent data collection and ideas to check against previously collected data.

---

[2] See the quotation from Hayes-Bautista in Charmaz (2000).

Box 10.1 Initial coding: line-by-line coding.

Excerpt 1,
I: (3) The next question is thinking about why, um, patients with brain injury might exhibit challenging behaviour and you've, you've kind of talked a bit about that, you know, the processes in the brain. Is there anything else you want to add to that?

Acknowledging multiple reasons	P-D: There's so many reasons why a patient might
Repeating all-inclusive	display challenging behaviour. Loss of identity,
euphemism –'challenging'	you know, loss, they suffer huge losses, they
Delineating reasons – stressing	might lose their family because of the change in
magnitude of losses: suffering	personality, families just can't cope with, you
rejection; identifying identity	know, this changing person. They might lose their
loss, family because of	children, they might lose their home, you know,
personality changes, children,	they'll lose um, lose their job. I think, I don't think
home, job	enough emphasis is placed on that fact that these
Losing one's life, way of being in	people have lost their life. And basically through
the world	that they have perhaps experienced a huge range,
Suffering massive loss; having	huge range of losses and because of their
alienated others	behaviour they may have alienated people so that
Misbehaving cloaks loss	there is just this massive aspect of loss that they all
Misreading behaviour (by staff)	have. And again, again I don't think that there are
	people that appreciate that, that they are doing it
Acting up reflects loss	because they are acting up, or they are doing it
	because they want something when in effect, you
Confronting loss constantly;	know, they might just be constantly thinking
surveying probable pasts	about how much they've lost. I mean um, well
Explaining all-encompassing loss	you know . . . patient, well . . . patient has lost
	everything she lost her, you know she had a flat
Being aware of devastating	with her, well she was engaged she had a, you
losses; Losing one's prior life	know, a really good job, fantastic social life. And
Having nothing left	she's got nothing now, and, you know, quite
	rightly so that, she's, you know, on days where
Comparing self with others;	she's feeling low and sees people going off doing
Explaining emotional response	things that she can't do. Her level of arousal is
Understanding the magnifying of	going to rise, so if you even say wait a minute to
small slights;	her, its important to her. And I think that's
Forgetting to place patient's	another thing that people forget it that, although
behaviour in context; staff	it might seem a petty small request or something
bifurcating patient's biography	small that. People forget that to them [patients]

(Continued)

Box 10.1 (*Cont'd*)

	that's, that's important to them and they haven't
Acknowledging lack of life	got much of a life, um (.) I do think that once
	people have been here a long time, I think some
Pointing out staff's overlooking	people do forget that these patients have lost
loss	everything. And quite frankly I think I'd probably
Putting self in patient's situation	want to be as awkward as I could if it meant that I
	would get somebody to talk to me. Um, if they
Understanding patient's	can't communicate, you know quite often they'll
frustration with varied causes	lose their ability to speak, you know, they're going
of loss	to get frustrated with that. If they've lost their
Connecting patient's losses with	ability to walk, you know its just so many, so
current mental health	many different aspects that could, you know, it
	can impact on their mental health if they had
	issues before, or they might, you know, they
	might become depressed (2). Its just so, so,
	physical issues, things that they can't do. You
Understanding loss of autonomy,	know, its somebody who was quite proud, you
dignity	know, quite an independent person who can't
Placing patient's anger in context	wash themselves, is going to get pissed off with it.
	Something that people don't, aren't, don't get a
Failing to grasp meanings of loss	grasp of through just working with patients every
Lacking empathy–staff	day. I don't think people really, I don't think the
	empathy is always there. . . .

The coding in Box 10.1 is a secondary analysis of data from a study of staff in hospital for people with brain impairment (Stewart, 2007). The interviewer aimed to discover which kinds of patient behaviour staff found to be troubling. In keeping with grounded theory logic, she adopted the staff's term, 'challenging behaviour', and asked questions to break open this institutional euphemism. She crafted well-designed questions to find out what challenging behaviour meant to the interview participants. Her open-ended interviewing style allowed interviewees to concentrate on what they saw as most significant while she simultaneously explored the properties of challenging behaviour and the conditions under which staff defined it.

Note that the codes in Box 10.1 use gerunds and demonstrate actions. The interview excerpt in Box 10.1 draws on three sources of actions: those of Participant D (P-D), her descriptions of actions of brain-injured patients in the hospital where she works, and her views of the actions of other people (staff) toward patients' actions. What is Participant D doing? The codes define her actions as 'acknowledging multiple reasons', 'repeating the all-inclusive euphemism, "challenging behaviour"', 'delineating reasons' for this behaviour, 'explaining all-encompassing loss' and 'putting self in patient's situation'. Participant D explains these patients' experience in codes such as 'suffering rejection', 'suffering massive loss', 'having nothing left' and 'being aware of devastating losses'. When she considers patients' challenging behaviour in the hospital, Participant D's statements and therefore the codes reveal another line of action such as 'misbehaving cloaks loss', 'misreading behaviour' (by staff), 'forgetting to place patient's behaviour in context', 'staff bifurcating patient's biography', 'failing to grasp meanings of loss' and 'lacking empathy' (for guidelines for coding see Charmaz, 2006; Corbin & Strauss, 2008). All these codes suggest areas that the researcher could develop and check in subsequent interviews or observations.

Might another analyst come up with different codes? Yes, our perspectives and social locations affect how we code. Different researchers coding the same data may generate new insights. After studying their initial codes, researchers can then treat their most compelling and frequent codes as *focused codes* to sort, synthesize and analyse large batches of data (Charmaz, 2006).

What does memo-writing involve?

Memo-writing is the pivotal analytic stage between coding and writing the first draft of a paper or chapter. Memo-writing occurs from the beginning of data collection and proceeds throughout the research process. Early memos are partial, tentative and exploratory, filled with empirical information to check and analytic questions to pursue (see the questions in the early sample memo below, 'Explaining All-Encompassing Loss'). Later memos are more precise, abstract, sophisticated and conceptually robust, and may demonstrate relationships between theoretical categories as well as analyse a single category such as becoming marginalized. By subjecting key codes to further analysis, grounded theorists probe their data and examine how these codes hold up as tentative categories. Further checks occur as grounded theorists seek increasingly specific data to test their emerging analyses of the category or categories they are developing.

Box 10.2 Sample Memo

Explaining All-Encompassing Loss

Explaining all encompassing loss means making explicit unknown or forgotten meanings of the magnitude of patients' loss. Explaining here means pointing out types of loss patients have experienced, delineating their extent, and making these losses known and understood. Explaining all-encompassing loss means taking the *patient's* perspective and looking at what is lost. Loss resides in the chasm between the life once lived and current institutional existence. Participant D points out,

(Continued)

Box 10.2 (*Cont'd*)

"I think, I don't think enough emphasis is placed on that fact that these people have *lost* their life. And basically through that they have perhaps experienced a huge range, huge range of losses and because of their behaviour they may have alienated people so that there is just this massive aspect of loss that they all have." Thus, loss can result in spiraling consequences. Awareness of losing one's life, one's way of being in the world causes patients enormous suffering that they may express through frustration, anger, and aggression, which leads to being rejected and further suffering, and subsequently more acting up. Misbehaving cloaks loss, and then, staff misread the patient's behavior. Conditions that exacerbate this process include the nature of the patient's impairment and its relative visibility, the extent to which it complicates daily life, and the institutional situation itself. To what extent does being subject to this situation impart messages that lapses in self-control are routine events and therefore desensitize patients as well as staff to troublesome behavior?

Explaining all-encompassing loss not only asks the listener to envision losses, but also to envision who a patient was before experiencing brain impairment. Thus, staff would gain a different image of the patient than that of the person they encounter in their daily work. Explaining links the past with the present and accounts for the present. (In contrast to Participant D's accounting for the present by looking at the past, Participant B considers impairment but concentrates on the present, not the magnitude of loss, nor the suffering it may cause.) Participant D adopts the role of the teacher who elucidates for the interviewer why patients act as they do. To what extent can or does she make her views known and heard? How does she deal with co-workers who fail to grasp these meanings of loss?

By explaining all-encompassing loss, Participant D presents herself as empathetic, insightful, and different – separate? – from co-workers. How does her empathy alter relationships with patients? How and when do her insights affect her work with patients? What, if any, are the implications of setting oneself apart from co-workers in this setting?

At every stage of memo-writing, grounded theorists analyse their data and thus move beyond description and summaries of data. Memo-writing advances comparative processes of comparing data with data, data with code, code with code, code with category, and category with category. Memo-writing also prompts a researcher to define the code, delineate its properties and to specify conditions when this code is or is not manifest. Note that the memo above specifies conditions and outlines how this code fits into an overall process that integrates other codes. Does the memo capture empirical reality?

Through memo-writing, researchers may also explicate research participants' implicit assumptions and show how the codes reveal them. Writing memos spurs making discoveries because researchers develop fleeting ideas and define phenomena that they had not noticed before coding. Several other memo-writing suggestions help:

1. *Title memos:* make sorting, synthesizing, and storing easy;
2. *Keep the analysis grounded:* construct definitions and properties of codes or categories from data;
3. *Show processes:* delineate conditions under which a code or category emerges, is maintained or changes;
4. *Include evidence:* insert data excerpts that generate or support a code or category; and
5. *Track ideas:* write memos whenever an idea arises.

Memos give grounded theorists an analytic understanding of processes, substance for papers and chapters, tentative categories to interrogate further through theoretical sampling, and material for future projects.

What Makes for a Better Quality Grounded Theory Study?

Similar to all forms of research, grounded theory studies vary in quality and unfortunately many published examples offer little more than a glorified description of an experience or phenomenon. In psychology, key tenets in determining the quality of qualitative research studies relate to the adaptation of the scientific canons of *validity, reliability* and *generalizability*.

Within grounded theory, Strauss and Corbin (1990, 1998) also guard against the unquestioning adherence to the three scientific canons as applied to quantitative research. They argue that these canons 'require redefinition in order to fit the realities of qualitative research and the complexities of social phenomena' (Strauss & Corbin, 1990, p. 250). To evaluate grounded theory studies, Strauss and Corbin pose questions about the data, research process and empirical grounding of the findings. Their questions relate to systematic and transparent handling of the data, the level and development of categories and processes, and the significance of any theoretical findings. Charmaz (2006) also highlights evaluative criteria for grounded theory studies, classifying the areas of *credibility, originality, resonance* and *usefulness*. Scholars can use these criteria to evaluate studies by Charmaz (1991), Qin and Lykes (2006) and Shrock and Padavic (2007). Yet, even within these useful frameworks, researchers' epistemological positions shape their different emphases on various criteria. Madill *et al.* (2000) have used an example of a grounded theory study to compare how different criteria may be applied when alternative epistemological positions are taken: post-positivism and constructivist. They conclude that research needs to be 'evaluated by the standards entailed by its own logic of justification' (Madill *et al.*, 2000, p. 17).

Future Directions for Grounded Theory

The increasing popularity of grounded theory since its conception in the late 1960s has naturally led to an evolution in terms of grounded theory's epistemological underpinnings, emphasis and methodology. Constructivist versions of grounded theory have been developed (see Charmaz, 2006), altering the emphasis of the approach from *discovery* of theory to *generation,* accepting the interplay and connectivity between the researched, researched and interpretations made. Moves towards pragmatism, pleuralism and mixed methods (Madill & Gough, 2008) have enabled grounded theorists to use other methodologies as a complement in order to address broad-ranging research questions. In addition, new frameworks for analysis and theory-building such as situational analysis (Clarke, 2003, 2005) and fractal concept analysis (Wasserman *et al.,* 2009) have assisted researchers in moving away from descriptive accounts. Without doubt, this new generation of grounded theorists will continue to develop grounded theory in interesting and innovative ways.

As with epistemology and emphasis, the forms of media suitable for grounded theory analysis have also evolved in recent times, providing researchers with alternatives to the commonly used interview method. Grounded theorists have used focus groups to generate material (Henwood & Pidgeon, 2003), reflective commentary of events using Interpersonal Process Recall (Rennie, 2005) and increasingly recognize that visual media may be a suitable form of data for qualitative researchers to analyse (Gleeson *et al.,* 2005). Within mental health research, these new directions alongside greater service user involvement throughout the entire research process provide not only challenges but opportunities to grounded theory researchers. It is an exciting time to engage in grounded theory research, not only to elucidate and situate the social and organizational processes service users experience, but to strengthen the connections between the academic and clinical worlds.

Acknowledgement

The authors would particularly like to thank Dr Inga Stewart, Senior Clinical Psychologist, for allowing us to use some of her interview data (with the participants' permission) for the worked examples in the coding and memo-writing sections of the chapter. It is very much appreciated.

References

Anderson, J. (2006). Well-suited partners: Psychoanalytic research and grounded theory. *Journal of Child Psychotherapy, 32,* 329–348.

Blumer, H. (1969). *Symbolic interactionism.* Englewood Cliffs, NJ: Prentice-Hall.

Bowen, G.A. (2008). Naturalistic inquiry and the saturation concept: A research note. *Qualitative Research, 8,* 137–152.

Boyd, T. & Gumley, A. (2007). An experiential perspective on persecutory paranoia: A grounded theory construction. *Psychology and Psychotherapy: Theory,* Research and Practice, *80,* 1–22.

Braun, V. & Clarke, V. (2006). Using thematic analysis in psychology. *Qualitative Research in Psychology, 3,* 77–102.

Burck, C. (2005). Comparing qualitative research methodologies for systemic research: The use of grounded theory, discourse analysis and narrative analysis. *Journal of Family Therapy, 27,* 237–262.

Charmaz, K. (1991). *Good days, bad days: The self in chronic illness and time.* New Brunswick, NJ: Rutgers University Press.

Charmaz, K. (2000). Teachings of Anselm Strauss: Remembrances and reflections. *Sociological Perspectives, 43,* S163–S174.

Charmaz, K. (2006). *Constructing grounded theory: A practical guide through qualitative analysis.* London: Sage.

Charmaz, K. (2008). Views from the margins: Voices, silences, and suffering. *Qualitative Research in Psychology, 5,* 7–18.

Charmaz, K. (2009). Shifting the grounds: Constructivist grounded theory methods for the twenty-first century. In J. Morse, P. Stern, J. Corbin, B. Bowers, K. Charmaz & A. Clarke. *Developing grounded theory: The second generation* (pp. 127–154). Walnut Creek, CA: Left Coast Press.

Charmaz, K. (in press). Grounded theory methods in social justice research. In N.K. Denzin & Y.E. Lincoln (Eds.)*Handbook of qualitative research* (4th edn). Thousand Oaks, CA: Sage.

Charmaz, K. & Rosenfeld, D. (2006). Reflections of the body, images of self: Visibility and invisibility in chronic illness and disability. In D.D. Waskul & P. Vannini (Eds.)*Body/embodiment: Symbolic interaction and the sociology of the body* (pp. 35–50). London: Ashgate.

Chiovitti, R.F. (2008). Nurses' meaning of caring with patients in acute psychiatric hospital settings: A grounded theory study. *International Journal of Nursing Studies, 45,* 203–223.

Clarke, A.E. (2003) Situational analysis: Grounded theory mapping after the postmodern turn. *Symbolic Interaction, 26,* 553–576.

Clarke, A.E. (2005). *Situational analysis: Grounded theory after the postmodern turn.* Thousand Oaks, CA: Sage.

Corbin, J.M. & Strauss, A.C. (2008). Basics of qualitative research: Techniques and procedures for developing grounded theory (3rd edn). Los Angeles, CA: Sage.

Frankel, Z. & Levitt, H.M. (2009). Clients' experiences of disengaged moments in psychotherapy: A grounded theory analysis. *Journal of Contemporary Psychotherapy, 39,* 171–186.

Glaser, B.G. (1978). *Theoretical sensitivity.* Mill Valley, CA: Sociology Press.

Glaser, B.G. (1992). *Basics of grounded theory analysis.* Mill Valley, CA: Sociology Press.

Glaser, B.G. (1998). *Doing grounded theory: Issues and discussions.* Mill Valley, CA: Sociology Press.

Glaser, B.G. & Strauss, A.L. (1967). *The discovery of grounded theory.* Chicago: Aldine.

Gleeson, K., Archer, L., Riley, S. & Frith, H. (2005). Visual methodologies. *Qualitative Research in Psychology, 2,* 187–198.

Henwood, K.L. & Pidgeon, N.F. (2003). Grounded theory in psychological research. In P. Camic, J. Rhodes & L. Yardley (Eds.) *Qualitative research in psychology: Expanding perspectives in methodology and design* (pp. 131–155). Washington, DC: APA Publications.

Homewood, E., Tweed, A., Cree, M. & Crossley, J. (2009). Becoming occluded: The transition to motherhood of women with post-natal depression. *Qualitative Research in Psychology, 6,* 1–17.

Karp, D. (1996). *Speaking of sadness: Depression, disconnection, and the meanings of illness.* New York: Oxford University Press.

Madill, A. & Gough, B. (2008). Qualitative research and its place in psychological science. *Psychological Methods, 13,* 254–271.

Madill, A., Jordan, A. & Shirley, C. (2000). Objectivity and reliability in qualitative analysis: Realist, contextualist and radical constructivist epistemologies. *British Journal of Psychology, 91,* 1–20.

Morse, J.M. (1995). The significance of saturation. *Qualitative Health Research, 5,* 147–149.

Noiseux, S. & Ricard, N. (2008). Recovery as perceived by people with schizophrenia, family members and health professionals: A grounded theory. *International Journal of Nursing Studies, 45,* 1148–1162.

Qin, D. & Lykes, M.B. (2006). Reweaving a fragmented self: A grounded theory of self-understanding among Chinese women students in the United States of America. *International Journal of Qualitative Studies in Education, 19,* 177–200.

Rennie, D.L. (2005). The grounded theory method: Application of a variant of its procedure of constant comparative analysis to psychotherapy research. In C.T. Fischer (Ed.) *Qualitative research methods for psychologists: Introduction through empirical studies* (pp. 59–78). London: Academic Press.

Rennie, D., Phillips, J.R. & Quartaro, G.K. (1988). Grounded theory: A promising approach to conceptualisation in psychology. *Canadian Psychology, 29,* 139–150.

Rose, D., Fleischmann, P. & Wykes, T. (2004). Consumers' views of electroconvulsive therapy: A qualitative analysis. *Journal of Mental Health, 13,* 285–293.

Schrock, D.P. & Padavic, I. (2007). Negotiating hegemonic masculinity in a batterer intervention program. *Gender and Society, 21,* 625–649.

Smith, J.A. (1996). Beyond the divide between cognition and discourse: Using interpretative phenomenological analysis in health psychology. *Psychology and Health, 11,* 261–271.

Stewart, I. (2007). Attributions regarding challenging behaviour within an acquired brain injury setting: A grounded theory analysis. Unpublished thesis: Leicester University.

Strauss, A. & Corbin, J. (1990). *Basics of qualitative research: Grounded theory procedures and techniques.* Newbury Park, CA: Sage.

Strauss, A. & Corbin, J. (1998). *Basics of qualitative research: Techniques and procedures for developing grounded theory* (2nd edn). Newbury Park, CA: Sage.

Suddaby, R. (2006). From the editors: What grounded theory is not. *Academy of Management Journal, 49,* 633–642.

Teram, E., Schachter, C.L. & Stalker, C.A. (2005). The case for integrating grounded theory and participatory action research: Empowering clients to inform professional practice. *Qualitative Health Research, 15,* 1129–1140.

Wasserman, J.A., Clair, J.M. & Wilson, K.L. (2009). Problematics of grounded theory: Innovations for developing an increasingly rigorous qualitative method. *Qualitative Research, 9,* 355–381.

Wilson, H.S. (1977). Limiting intrusion: Social control of outsiders in a healing community. *Nursing Research, 26,* 105–111.

Wuest, J., Ford-Gilboe, M., Merritt-Gray, M. & Lemire, S. (2006). Using grounded theory to generate a theoretical understanding of the effects of child custody policy on women's health promotion in the context of intimate partner violence. *Health Care for Women International,* *27*, 490–512.

Further reading and useful website

Charmaz, K. (2006). *Constructing grounded theory: A practical guide through qualitative analysis.* London: Sage.

Corbin, J. & Strauss, A. (2008) *Basics of qualitative research techniques and procedures for developing grounded theory* (3rd edn). Los Angeles: Sage.

Grounded Theory Institute: www.groundedtheory.com.

11

Discourse Analysis

Eugenie Georgaca and Evrinomy Avdi

Discourse analysis, as an approach to studying psychological phenomena, developed out of the 'turn to language' in social psychology in the 1970s and 1980s and the emergence of social constructionism. Although its main developments have taken place in social psychology, over the last two decades it has been increasingly used in the fields of clinical psychology, counselling psychology and psychotherapy, where it is usually associated with critical approaches.

Description

Discourse analysis is a broad and diverse field, including a variety of approaches to the study of language, which derive from different scientific disciplines and utilize various analytical practices (Wetherell *et al.*, 2001a,b). In a broad sense, discourses are defined as *systems of meaning* that are related to the interactional and wider socio-cultural context and operate regardless of the speakers' intentions. Discourse analysis examines language in use, rather than the psychological phenomena such as attitudes, memory or emotions which are traditionally presumed to underlie talk and be revealed through it.

In discourse analysis, language is examined in terms of *construction* and *function*; that is, language is considered a means of constructing, rather than mirroring, reality. Language is also considered a form of *social action*; people use language to achieve certain interpersonal goals (e.g., attribute responsibility, refute blame, etc.) in specific interactional contexts. Discourse analysis, therefore, examines how certain issues are constructed in people's accounts and the *variability* in these accounts, and explores the *rhetorical* aspects and the functions of talk in the *context* of the ongoing interaction

Qualitative Research Methods in Mental Health and Psychotherapy: A Guide for Students and Practitioners, First Edition. Edited by D. Harper and A.R. Thompson.
© 2012 John Wiley & Sons, Ltd. Published 2012 by John Wiley & Sons, Ltd.

(Potter & Wetherell, 1987). Discourses entail *subject positions*, which speakers take up when they employ language, and this has fundamental consequences both for the sense of self and experience of the speakers, and for the actions they are entitled and expected to perform. Furthermore, there is a mutual relationship between discourses and *institutions*; discourses are produced and disseminated through institutional practices and they in turn legitimize and maintain these practices. Finally, discourses are wrapped up with *power*, because they make available certain versions of reality and personhood, whilst marginalizing alternative knowledges and associated practices. Discourse analysis examines the ways in which discourses permeate talk and other kinds of texts. Discourse analysis also involves looking at the effects of discourses on, for example, how we experience ourselves and relate to each other. These discourses may reproduce or challenge culturally dominant ways of understanding the world, and, in turn, thus reproduce or challenge dominant institutions and the particular kinds of social order (e.g., Parker, 1992).

Historical Origins and Influences

Discourse analysis is closely linked to the 'turn to language' and the emergence of social constructionism. A specifically discursive approach emerged in psychology in the mid 1980s, mainly in the United Kingdom, and since its inception took shape in two distinct yet partly overlapping trends. One approach, which was later termed *discursive psychology*, drew upon developments in linguistic philosophy, semiology, the sociology of scientific knowledge, ethnomethodology, conversation analysis and rhetorical work in psychology (Wiggins & Potter, 2008). Discursive psychology is primarily concerned with discursive practices, that is to say, with the ways in which speakers in everyday and institutional settings negotiate meaning, reality, identity and responsibility. Another trend, subsequently termed *Foucauldian discourse analysis*, drew upon post-structuralist theorists, such as Foucault, Barthes and Derrida, cultural studies and social theory, and was informed by feminism and Marxism (Arribas-Ayllon & Walkerdine, 2008; Burman & Parker, 1993). Foucauldian discourse analysis focuses on discursive resources and examines the ways in which discourses construct objects and subjects, and create, in this way, certain versions of reality, society and identity as well as maintaining certain practices and institutions (Willig, 2008).

Key Epistemological Assumptions

Discourse analysis is a social constructionist approach. For *social constructionism*, reality and identity are systematically constructed and maintained through systems of meaning and through social practices. In terms of epistemology, many discourse theorists adopt a *relativist* view; they assume that there exist no objective grounds on which the truth of claims can be proven and propose that the value of knowledge should be evaluated according to other criteria, such as its applicability, usefulness and clarity (Potter, 1996). However, others claim that relativism does not allow for a position from which social critique and action can be developed and adopt a *critical realist position*; they acknowledge that knowledge is always mediated by social processes but propose that underlying enduring structures do exist and that these can be known through their effects (Parker, 2002). These debates are discussed in more detail in Chapter 7.

Research Questions

Given its emphasis on construction and function, discourse analysis neither asks questions about nor makes claims about the reality of people's lives or experiences but examines the ways in which reality and experience are constructed through social and interpersonal processes. In the field of psychotherapy, discourse analytic studies have investigated:

1. The transformation of meaning in the course of therapy;
2. The negotiation of agency, responsibility and blame between therapist and clients;
3. The role of the therapist in shaping clients' accounts;
4. Power and resistance; and
5. The role of hegemonic discourses in shaping clients' problems and the solutions to them (for review see Avdi, 2008; Avdi & Georgaca, 2007, 2009; Georgaca & Avdi, 2009).

Mental health topics investigated by discourse analytic studies include:

1. Critical examination of clinical categories through tracing their historical trajectory (e.g., Blackman, 2001; Hepworth, 1999) or deconstructing their underlying assumptions (e.g., Georgaca, 2000; Gillett, 1997);
2. Analysing the effects of discourses in shaping experiences and views of service users (e.g., Burns & Gavey, 2004; Swann & Ussher, 1995);
3. Examination of the ways in which professionals construct clinical cases and justify their practices (e.g., Griffiths, 2001; Stevens & Harper, 2007);
4. How mental illness is constructed in public texts, including policy, media and cultural texts (e.g., Bilić & Georgaca, 2007; Harper, 2004; for a review see Harper, 2006).

Appropriate Data

Discourse analysis can be applied to any kind of *text* (i.e., to anything that has meaning; Parker, 2002), although most studies analyse written or spoken language. Discourse analysis has been used to analyse both naturally occurring and research-generated texts. In the field of mental health and psychotherapy, studies published to date have used interviews with individuals with mental health problems, interviews with mental health professionals, transcripts of professional interactions and psychotherapy sessions, newspaper reports, cultural texts and policy documents.

Regarding *data sampling and size*, discourse analyses often rely on relatively small numbers of participants and/or texts, in part because analysis is very labour-intensive and large amounts of data would be prohibitive. The appropriate amount of data depends on the specific research question and the depth of the analysis conducted, but as a rule of thumb eight to twenty interviews or four to eight focus group discussions should provide adequate material for a publishable study.

Involvement of Research Participants and Mental Health Service Users

Discourse analysis tends to fall short of involving participants in the research process, largely because of its interpretative nature. The simplest level of participation, *participant validation*, which is used in some forms of qualitative inquiry, is not a process commonly practised in discourse analytic studies (for a discussion see Harper, 2003). Discourse analysis relies on an assumption that individuals are both positioned by discourses (of which they may not be fully aware) and use them (although not necessarily intentionally). It does not therefore make sense to ask research participants to validate something of which they may not be fully conscious (Coyle, 2000).

However, other researchers have claimed that discourse analysis can be used to enable research participants to become aware of the ways in which they are positioned through discourse. It has been argued, for example, that through highlighting the role of discourses in shaping experience, subjectivity and practices, discourse analysis could be useful in deconstructing taken for granted assumptions and in increasing the reflexivity of mental health professionals, thus contributing to more competent and empowering professional practices (e.g., Kogan & Brown, 1998). Similarly, Willig (1999) suggests that the process of conducting a discourse analytic study can be used either 'therapeutically', as a way of shifting participants' subjectivities through reflexively examining their positioning, or as a form of consciousness raising, whereby participants explore the ways in which they have been constrained by certain discourses. In this way, discourse analysis can be used by socially oppressed and marginalized groups, including mental health service users, as a tool for empowerment, through exploring the subtle ways in which they have been subjugated by dominant symbolic systems and practices (Willig, 1999). This suggestion moves beyond participant validation to forms of *collaborative and/or user-led research* (see Chapter 4) which is a direction in which research in mental health and psychotherapy should be moving (Harper, 2008). Nevertheless, the study by Armes (2009) is the only user-led discourse analytic study to date of which we are aware.

Use of the Method and Example

There is no wide agreement regarding the process of discourse analysis, although several guides to conducting discourse analytic research (Billig, 1997; Potter & Wetherell, 1987; Wiggins & Potter, 2008) and to analysing discourse (Parker, 1992; Potter, 2003) have been published. The steps in conducting a discourse analytic study broadly include devising a research question, gaining access and consent, collecting data, transcribing, reading, coding, analysis, validation, writing and application. In this section we concentrate on the process of analysing discourse, whereby we adopt an overall critical Foucauldian perspective, but for the actual micro-analysis we utilize the analytical tools of discursive psychology (Willig, 2008). Our aim is to introduce the basic notions and illustrate the main analytic practices used in discourse analysis, rather than offer a set of fixed procedures.

Analysis begins with transcription, which necessarily entails a degree of interpretation (O'Connell & Kowal, 1995). Following transcription, several close readings and an initial coding is performed, which involves a selection of a corpus of extracts deemed relevant to the research question. This preliminary analysis leads the researcher to immerse him or herself in the data and begin to develop a sense of the flavour and the functions of the text. Analysis proper follows, which we present in terms of several inter-related levels, as applied to a brief extract from a family therapy session.

The extract presented is drawn from a family therapy session that took place in a Community Mental Health Centre in Greece[1] and has been presented in more detail in Avdi (2005). The family (consisting of John, Anne and son Tom, aged 3.5 years) visited the service because of concerns regarding Tom's development; Tom had been previously given a diagnosis of autism, psychosis and learning disability by different professionals. In the following extract, drawn from the beginning of the first session, Anne explains how the parents gradually came to realize that there was a problem.

Extract[2]

1 Anne: he started making some movements, that is he started to say ah very intensely <u>aaaah</u>

2 he started to make these movements [*makes hand-flapping movements*], he started to hop and to

---

[1] In line with the Centre's usual practice, all family therapy sessions were audio-recorded and consent was obtained from the family for the use of transcribed material for research and teaching purposes. All names used here are pseudonyms.

[2] Transcription notation: underlining = added emphasis; (.) = brief pause; (...) = part of the text omitted.

3 clap his hands

4 Therapist: did these remind you of anything?

5 Anne: they didn't remind us of anything because we didn't know anything about such matters,

6 but we definitely thought that something was not quite right

7 Therapist: did they remind you of a child younger than Tom? because usually this is the sort of

8 hand clapping that babies do

9 Anne: no it wasn't that sort of clapping (.) this is the sort of hand-clapping (.) not like the children

10 to whom we say 'clap your hands' (.) Tom does it when he is very pleased, that is, he sees a

11 picture and he claps, he does this thing, moves his hands like this (.) he goes round and round

12 sometimes, around himself, it is not the sort of clapping that shows us that he is a child (.) to me it

13 was indication that something was wrong, it is not the clapping of a child (. . .) we could see

14 Tom did not say anything any more, he didn't even say hello, nothing, he did nothing, and these

15 things he does they became more intense, that is, he started saying aaah more intensely, the

16 hand-clapping became more intense, he started seeing some pictures, not all pictures, and to hop

17 Therapist: what pictures was it usually?

18 Anne: oh it makes no difference what the picture is, it could be just a line, for example, we had

19 this drawing pad the other day it had a paintbrush and something else on, I cannot remember

20 exactly what, and he liked it a lot and he started hopping around

21 Therapist: did it have colours? was it a drawing?

22 Tom: eeeeee

23 Therapist: what is his favourite picture?

24 Anne: I cannot say that he has a specific picture, it is a thing of the moment, he may get hold of a

25 magazine and look at it and choose one picture that he likes from the whole magazine and start to

26 hop around (. . .) I get frustrated in the sense that I don't know how to react, what I should do,

27 should I take the book off him so that he stops making these movements, I am thinking how to

28 stop these movements he makes, because, that is, I think 'you go out, they see Tom', er, your life

29 becomes different afterwards

Level 1: Language as constructive: Discourses

A basic assumption underlying discourse analysis relates to the constructive aspect of language; that is, the assumption that texts construct the objects to which they refer, that is to say, they create specific versions of the phenomena and processes they set out to describe. Accordingly, the first step in the analysis is to examine the various ways in which the objects under study are constructed in the specific text. We examine all instances where the object is mentioned or implied, and focus on the variability in the constructions.

The object under study in the example concerns the negotiation of the problem that takes place in the clinical dialogue. We briefly examine the mother's and the therapist's constructions in turn. Anne produces a list of Tom's behaviours which includes vocalizations, movements with a compulsive quality, general apathy and lack of speech. These behaviours are represented as typical of Tom, unusual (lines 9, 10), bizarre and inexplicable (lines 9–16, 24–29), an indication that something is wrong (lines 12, 13) and something to be managed, stopped and concealed from others (lines 26–29). The therapist's questions introduce a different interpretative frame regarding the problematic behaviours; her first question implies that the behaviours could be understood in the context of Anne's previous experience, a construction further developed in her second utterance (lines 7, 8), where she presents, in an apparently normalizing manner, Tom's handclapping as part of a developmental course. Moreover, through her next questions (lines 17, 23), the therapist elaborates the notion that there may be a pattern, and therefore a meaning, in Tom's seemingly bizarre behaviours, thus constructing the problem as meaningful action rather than a meaningless symptom.

After establishing the different modes of the object's construction, we broaden our focus to locate these constructions within culturally available systems of meaning, that is to say, discourses. This is the first step towards linking interaction with ideology.

In this brief extract one can begin to discern the systems of meaning from which the parents and the therapist draw in their talk. Anne lists Tom's behaviours without associating them with Tom's inner world or interactional context (lines 1–3, 9–16, 24–26) and therefore these behaviours take on, we would argue, the quality of symptoms. In Anne's talk, therefore, the problem and Tom's identity can be seen to be primarily constructed in terms of a *medical discourse*. One of the features of the medical discourse is that it implicates the existence of a specific diagnosable condition, clearly located inside the person (in this case the child), which has a given (presumably organic) aetiology, prognosis and treatment. As we have already argued, language creates the objects it refers to and constructions are associated with sets of meanings as well as institutions and practices. Given the family's previous contact with professionals, it is not surprising that the behaviours (or symptoms) they use in describing their child are commonly associated with contemporary definitions of autism. Moreover, in comparing (lines 9–17) Tom's clapping with 'that sort of handclapping', Anne discursively creates a 'normal' type of handclapping, which the therapist is supposed to recognize, and which forms the basis with which comparisons are made. The notion that a normal range of children's behaviours can be defined is part of a *discourse of normal development*.

This discourse is associated with specific bodies of knowledge, such as developmental psychology, and with health care and educational practices that define what a normal child is expected to be able to do, when and how, assess these behaviours and treat children that deviate. In this framework, difference is generally framed in terms of deficiency or abnormality (Urwin, 1985). The discourse of normal development has been criticized for abstracting, reifying and privileging the notion of a prototypical genderless child, beyond context and culture (Burman, 2008) and for incorporating the assumption that parents, and particularly mothers, are responsible for promoting the emotional and intellectual health of their infant (Urwin, 1985).

In the last part of the extract Anne expresses her concerns about managing Tom's differentness (lines 27–29). Anne's concern regarding Tom *looking* different in conjunction with comparisons of Tom with 'normal children' (lines 9–16) can all be seen to be associated with a *disability discourse*. This discourse has associations of deficiency, locates the disabled person as Other and raises issues concerning the management of differentness, deviance and stigma (e.g., Avdi *et al.*, 2000). The therapist, on the other hand, through her questions that seek to associate Tom's behaviours with some meaningful internal state or treat them as meaningful responses within a certain context, is arguably deploying a *psychological/interpretative discourse*, which asserts that behaviour is always meaningful, even though this meaning may not be immediately apparent.

Level 2: Language as functional: Rhetorical strategies

A second level of analysis examines the dynamics of interaction; that is, the ways in which the participants' use of language and management of the interaction serve interpersonal functions (e.g., renouncement of an unwanted identity, attribution of responsibility, allocation of blame, etc.). Here we examine how accounts are organized and the rhetorical strategies speakers use in order to present their version as credible and themselves as objective, reliable and rational. In terms of the function of talk, we examine a speaker's utterance in relation to the discursive context in which it is produced; that is, what came before and what follows. We also examine the function that the deployment of specific discourses has on the unfolding interaction. Variability is a key feature of discourse use, as different discourses are used by the same speaker in different contexts, in order to serve varied discursive functions. A concept relevant here is the notion of the participants' *discursive agenda*, a notion that refers to the effects each participant's talk has on the overall interaction. The agenda of each participant can be deduced only after the detailed analysis of the function of his or her talk.

We briefly outline some hypotheses regarding action orientation (i.e., the possible functions of the speakers' utterances in the context of the particular interaction) by examining the first part of the extract. In her description of the problem, Anne uses various strategies that render her account credible and objective; for example, she provides a vivid and detailed description of Tom's symptoms and her account is structured so as to suggest that what is being described is a true and accurate version of reality, objectively represented by an unbiased and disinterested narrator (lines

1–3, 9–16, 18–21) (Potter, 1996). The therapist, in asking 'Did these remind you of anything?', asks for Anne's associations regarding Tom's behaviours, inviting her to attribute meaning to them; this intervention can be seen to subtly subvert the medical discourse, by challenging the view that the behaviours Anne describes have a single fixed meaning, shared by the speakers. Anne does not accept this invitation and her next utterance (lines 5, 6) can be read as furthering her aim to prove that that there is indeed an objective problem: she claims that initially they (here she includes her husband, thus increasing the persuasive power of her account) did not see Tom's behaviours for what they truly were (i.e., symptoms of autism), as they were naïve non-experts, although they could still see that something was wrong. Thus, Tom's difficulties are constructed as observable and objective facts, clearly obvious even to non-experts. Given that this exchange takes place during the family's first contact with the service, it could be argued that the parents are advocating for their child and attempting to convince professionals that there is a problem serious enough to warrant access to services. Next, the therapist introduces the notion that Tom's behaviours are like the actions of a young baby; this is an interesting intervention, as it both accepts the parents' view (i.e., that something is wrong) *and* reframes it as something that Tom can grow out of. This intervention is fairly typical in postmodern therapies, whereby restricting meanings are relativized without, however, rendering the therapist's account as the only valid perspective (e.g., Kogan & Gale, 1997).

The participants' agendas cannot be inferred from such a brief extract, although some indications of their overall effect on the interaction can be discerned. Anne's talk could be described as an attempt to convince experts of the reality of the problem, so that the family gains access to services, whilst refuting any possible accusations of blame, given that parents who attend services for their children may feel that they will be held responsible for their child's problems by professionals. Correspondingly, the therapist's discursive agenda seems to be that of destabilizing the dominance of the diagnostic discourse; the therapist's persistent attempts to attribute meaning to Tom's actions could be interpreted as an example of this.

Level 3: Positioning

Another important notion in the analysis is that of subject positions; that is, the identities made relevant through specific ways of talking (Davies & Harré, 1990). It is a notion that can be approached analytically on two levels: in relation to the specifics of the interaction and to wider discourses. First, in a particular interaction when participants speak, are addressed to or are spoken about, they are positioned in specific ways. Questions we raise at this level of analysis are: Who speaks? In whose name do they speak? Who do they address? Who do they speak for? Different positions entail differing degrees of accountability and can have a variety of functions (e.g., to distance the speaker from what is being said, to endow what is being said with authority, etc.). Secondly, discourses entail specific subject positions and, when participants draw upon certain discourses, they are positioned and call upon others to be positioned accordingly. The diagnostic discourse employed, for example, determines a pathological subject position for Tom. His actions are represented as conveying little meaning and being outside his control. Agency is attributed to the symptoms, represented as the manifestation of an underlying condition, abstracted from Tom and the context of his life, yet projected within him. Tom is positioned as someone fundamentally different from normal children, hovering somewhere between subjectivity and objectivity and he thus becomes the object of others' talk rather than a subject. This positioning is evident in the actual interaction, where Tom is talked about but not talked to, and when he participates in the conversation (line 23) he is not further involved in it.

In summarizing the above, analysis relies on the notions of discourse, action orientation and subject positioning, and these levels are often performed simultaneously and in conjunction. The following two levels examine the effects that discourse choice has on action and subjectivity, link the text with the wider social context and should follow the exhaustive micro-analysis of the text.

Level 4: Practices, institutions and power

There is a close mutual relationship between discourses and practices; dominant discourses, which become taken for granted, support and enable social and institutional practices, which in turn maintain them. The analytical questions here concern the role of the specific discourses used in maintaining or challenging dominant institutions and practices. This brings forth considerations of power, often considered in terms of the dominance of certain discourses, and resistance, which can take the form of clandestine use of discourses, refusal to take up the positions implied by dominant discourses or development and use of counter-discourses. With regards to this level of analysis, in the extract presented one could examine the effects of dominant discourses on the way in which the family's problems have been constituted as well as on the suggested ways of managing or resolving the problems. It would also be possible to investigate the interplay of power and resistance that takes place between therapist and parents in the clinical dialogue.

Level 5: Subjectivity

This last level of analysis concerns the effects of discourse on subjectivity. The adoption of the subject positions entailed in specific discourses has repercussions for the way individuals think, feel and experience themselves. Here we attempt to reconstitute what it means to be a person located in particular discourses. This level of analysis could explore the effects of positioning Tom in terms of the discourse of autism on his subjectivity and relationships.

Quality Criteria

With the recent proliferation of discourse analysis in the social sciences, several sets of fairly diverse quality criteria specific to discourse analysis have been published (Antaki et al., 2003; Burman, 2004; Potter & Wetherell, 1987). Chapter 16 includes generic criteria that could be used but, as a number of authors have suggested that qualitative researchers should identify evaluative criteria that are consistent with their epistemological assumptions and method, we note here those that we consider most useful and relevant for discourse analysts:

1. *Internal coherence* refers to the crafting of a consistent account of the data.
2. *Rigour* is achieved through attention to inconsistency and diversity, analysing deviant cases in order to delimit the applicability of data, and providing richness of detail.
3. The presentation of the research process should be *transparent and situated*, through the detailed explication of all the stages of the research process and the grounding of the analysis in extracts, so that the reader can judge both the quality of the findings and the relationship between the findings and the context of their generation.
4. *Reflexivity* is the overarching principle of constructionist studies; researchers should be attentive both to their role in the generation of research data and to the nature of the knowledge produced through the research, and should discuss these in the published study.
5. A final criterion for the quality of discourse analytic studies is their *usefulness* both theoretically, in terms of providing new insights, enhancing existing research and generating new questions, and in terms of their real world application.

Application

Discourse analysis has had a double impact: (i) it has shifted the focus from psychological phenomena to interpersonal processes and sociocultural systems of meaning, and (ii) it has been used to deconstruct dominant categories in psychology, by showing their historically located and socially constructed nature, and therefore to open spaces for alternative understandings (Coyle, 2000; Willig, 1999).

In the field of psychotherapy, discourse analyses have underscored its interactional nature and the active role of the therapist, and this can potentially promote therapist reflexivity. Discourse analytic studies of psychotherapy range from demonstrating the interactional processes through which psychotherapy is implemented, thus enhancing clinical work, to demonstrating how psychotherapy operates as an institution for the regulation of subjectivity, thus operating to deconstruct dominant psychotherapeutic assumptions and challenge psychotherapeutic practices (Avdi & Georgaca, 2007). In the field of mental health, studies attempt to deconstruct dominant categories and practices, by rendering visible the historical and cultural processes that have produced them, highlight the constraining effects dominant discourses have for people subjected to them and open the way for alternative, more empowering concepts and practices (Harper, 1995; Parker et al., 1995).

In summary, although discourse analytic findings do not lead to direct implemen-tation, they can inform novel interventions, especially those that oppose dominant understandings and practices (Harper, 2006).

Conclusions

Over the last two decades much discourse analytic work has been carried out in the field of psychotherapy but it has been more limited in the fields of psychopathology and serious mental distress. This may be because these studies of psychotherapy are linked with the recent emergence of postmodern trends in psychotherapeutic practice (McNamee & Gergen, 1992; Parker, 1999) – trends that are much less evident in mental health research as a result of the continued dominance of the medical model and the associated conservatism of this field.

Discourse analytic work has shifted the attention of psychological research to the interpersonal and social domains and has examined:

1. The interactional nature of professional practices, such as psychotherapy, diagnosis, case conferences;
2. The contingent, historically situated nature of dominant concepts and categories; and
3. The impact of these categories and associated practices on individuals who are subjected to them.

In this sense, discourse analysts, more than other researchers in mental health, have been on the critical edge, politically engaged and committed to critique and social change. Although we recognize that the more critical, deconstructive discourse analytic studies may be experienced as too far removed from the concerns clinicians face in their everyday work, we would still argue that critical work is the distinctive mark and the most important contribution that discourse analysis can make to mental health research (Avdi & Georgaca, 2007). Pursuing critical discourse analytic work with an aim of making a difference in the field would require: (i) emphasis on the links between research, implementation and interventions; (ii) alliances of discourse researchers with mental health service users and critical professionals; and (iii) tactical use of the findings through using multiple forms of dissemination and consultation (see also Harper, 2006).

References

Antaki, C., Billig, M., Edwards, D. & Potter, J. (2003). Discourse analysis means doing analysis: A critique of six analytic shortcomings. *Discourse Analysis Online.* Retrieved 20 April 2005 from http://www.shu.ac.uk/daol/articles/v1/n1/a1/antaki2002002-paper.html.

Armes, D.G. (2009). Mission informed discursive tactics of British mental health service-user/survivor movement (BSUSM) resistance to formalization pressures accompanying contractual relationships with purchasing authorities. *Journal of Mental Health, 18*(4), 344–352.

Arribas-Ayllon, M. & Walkerdine, W. (2008). Foucauldian discourse analysis. In C. Willig & W. Stainton-Rogers (Eds.) *The Sage handbook of qualitative research in psychology* (pp. 91–108). London: Sage.

Avdi, E. (2005). Discursively negotiating a pathological identity in the clinical dialogue: Discourse analysis of a family therapy. *Psychology and Psychotherapy: Theory, Research and Practice, 78,* 493–511.

Avdi, E. (2008). Analysing talk in the talking cure: Conversation, discourse and narrative analyses of psychoanalytic psychotherapy. *European Psychotherapy, 8,* 69–88.

Avdi, E. & Georgaca, E. (2007). Discourse analysis and psychotherapy: A critical review. *European Journal of Psychotherapy and Counselling, 9* (2), 157–176.

Avdi, E. & Georgaca, E. (2009). Narrative and discursive approaches to the analysis of subjectivity in psychotherapy. *Social and Personality Psychology Compass, 3* (5), 654–670.

Avdi, E., Griffin, C. & Brough, S. (2000). Parents' constructions of professional knowledge, expertise and authority during assessment and diagnosis of their child for an autistic spectrum disorder. *British Journal of Medical Psychology, 73,* 327–338.

Bilić, B. & Georgaca, E. (2007). Representations of 'mental illness' in Serbian newspapers: A critical discourse analysis. *Qualitative Research in Psychology, 4,* 167–186.

Billig, M. (1997). Rhetorical and discursive analysis: How families talk about the Royal Family. In N. Hayes (Ed.) *Doing qualitative analysis in psychology* (pp. 39–54). Hove: Psychology Press.

Blackman, L. (2001). *Hearing voices: Embodiment and experience.* London: Free Association Books.

Burman, E. (2004). Discourse analysis means analysing discourse: Some comments on Antaki, Billig, Edwards & Potter 'Discourse analysis means doing analysis: A critique of six analytic shortcomings'. *Discourse Analysis Online.* Retrieved 20 April 2005 from http://www.shu.ac.uk/daol/articles/open/2003/003/burman2003003-t.html.

Burman, E. (2008). *Deconstructing developmental psychology* (2nd edn). London: Routledge.

Burman, E. & Parker, I. (Eds.) (1993). *Discourse analytic research.* London: Routledge.

Burns, M. & Gavey, N. (2004). 'Healthy weight' at what cost? 'Bulimia' and a discourse of weight control. *Journal of Health Psychology, 9* (4), 549–565.

Coyle, A. (2000). Discourse analysis. In G.M. Breakwell, S. Hammond & C. Fife-Schaw (Eds.) *Research methods in psychology* (2nd edn, pp. 251–268). London: Sage.

Davies, B. & Harré, R. (1990). 'Positioning': The discursive production of selves. *Journal for the Theory of Social Behaviour, 20,* 43–63.

Georgaca, E. (2000). Reality and discourse: A critical analysis of the category of 'delusions'. *British Journal of Medical Psychology, 73,* 227–242.

Georgaca, E. & Avdi, E. (2009). Evaluating the talking cure: The contribution of narrative, discourse and conversation analysis to psychotherapy assessment. *Qualitative Research in Psychology, 6,* 233–247.

Gillett, G. (1997). A discursive account of multiple personality disorder. *Philosophy, Psychiatry and Psychology, 4,* 213–222.

Griffiths, L. (2001). Categorising to exclude: The discursive construction of cases in community mental health teams. *Sociology of Health and Illness, 23,* 678–700.

Harper, D. (2003). Developing a critically reflexive position using discourse analysis. In L. Finlay & B. Gough (Eds.) *Reflexivity: A practical guide for researchers in health and social sciences* (pp. 78–92). Oxford: Blackwell.

Harper, D. (2006). Discourse analysis. In M. Slade & S. Priebe (Eds.)*Choosing methods in mental health research: Mental health research from theory to practice* (pp. 47–67). London: Routledge.

Harper, D. (2008). Clinical psychology. In C. Willig & W. Stainton-Rogers (Eds.)*The Sage handbook of qualitative research in psychology* (pp. 430–454). London: Sage.

Harper, D.J. (1995). Discourse analysis and 'mental health'. *Journal of Mental Health, 4,* 347–357.

Harper, D.J. (2004). Storying policy: Constructions of risk in proposals to reform UK mental health legislation. In B. Hurwitz, V. Skultans & T. Greenhalgh (Eds.)*Narrative research in health and illness* (pp. 397–413). London: BMA Books.

Hepworth, J. (1999). *The social construction of anorexia.* London: Sage.

Kogan, S.M. & Brown, A.C. (1998). Reading against the lines: Resisting foreclosure in therapy. *Family Process, 37,* 495–512.

Kogan, S.M. & Gale, J.E. (1997). Decentering therapy: Textual analysis of a narrative therapy session. *Family Process, 36,* 101–126.

McNamee, S. & Gergen, K.J. (Eds.) (1992). *Therapy as social construction.* London: Sage.

O'Connell, D.C. & Kowal, S. (1995). Basic principles of transcription. In J.A. Smith, R. Harré & L. Van Langenhove (Eds.)*Rethinking methods in psychology* (pp. 93–105). London: Sage.

Parker, I. (1992). *Discourse dynamics: Critical analysis for social and individual psychology.* London: Routledge.

Parker, I. (Ed.) (1999). *Deconstructing psychotherapy.* London: Sage.

Parker, I. (2002). *Critical discursive psychology.* Basingstoke: Palgrave.

Parker, I., Georgaca, E., Harper, D., McLaughlin, T. & Stowell-Smith, M. (1995). *Deconstructing psychopathology.* London: Sage.

Potter, J. (1996). *Representing reality: Discourse, rhetoric and social construction.* London: Sage.

Potter, J. (2003). Discourse analysis and discursive psychology. In P.M. Camic, J.E. Rhodes & L. Yardley (Eds.) *Qualitative research in psychology: Expanding perspectives in methodology and design* (pp. 73–94). Washington: American Psychological Association.

Potter, J. & Wetherell, M. (1987). *Discourse and social psychology: Beyond attitudes and behaviour.* London: Sage.

Stevens, P. & Harper, D.J. (2007). Professional accounts of electroconvulsive therapy: A discourse analysis. *Social Science and Medicine, 64,* 1475–1486.

Swann, C.J. & Ussher, J.M. (1995). A discourse analytic approach to women's experience of premenstrual syndrome. *Journal of Mental Health, 4,* 359–367.

Urwin, C. (1985). Constructing motherhood: The persuasion of normal development. In C. Steedman, C. Urwin & V. Walkerdine (Eds.)*Language, gender and childhood* (pp. 164–202). London: Routledge and Kegan Paul.

Wetherell, M., Taylor, S. & Yates, S.J. (Eds.) (2001a). *Discourse theory and practice: A reader.* London: Sage.

Wetherell, M., Taylor, S. & Yates, S.J. (Eds.) (2001b). *Discourse as data: A guide for analysis.* London: Sage.

Wiggins, S. & Potter, J. (2008). Discursive psychology. In C. Willig & W. Stainton-Rogers (Eds.)*The Sage handbook of qualitative research in psychology* (pp. 73–90). London: Sage.

Willig, C. (Ed.) (1999). *Applied discourse analysis: Social and psychological interventions.* Buckingham: Open University Press.

Willig, C. (2008). *Introducing qualitative research in psychology: Adventures in theory and method* (2nd edn). Maidenhead: Open University Press.

Further reading

General introductions to discourse analysis

Wetherell, M., Taylor, S. & Yates, S.J. (Eds.) (2001a). *Discourse theory and practice: A reader.* London: Sage. [Advanced overview of theories and approaches to discourse]

Wetherell, M., Taylor, S. & Yates, S.J. (Eds.) (2001b). *Discourse as data: A guide for analysis.* London: Sage. [Advanced but very clear overview of different approaches to discourse analysing data]

Willig, C. (2008). *Introducing qualitative research in psychology: Adventures in theory and method* (2nd edn). Maidenhead: Open University Press. [Very clear introductory chapters on the two main trends of discourse analysis]

Overviews of discourse analysis in psychotherapy and mental health

Avdi, E. & Georgaca, E. (2007). Discourse analysis and psychotherapy: A critical review. *European Journal of Psychotherapy and Counselling, 9*(2), 157–176.

Harper, D. (2006). Discourse analysis. In M. Slade & S. Priebe (Eds.) *Choosing methods in mental health research: Mental health research from theory to practice* (pp. 47–67). London: Routledge.

12

Narrative Psychology

Michael Murray and Sally Sargeant

Description of Method

Narrative psychology starts with the assumption that in everyday life people organize their interpretations of reality in the form of narratives. These narratives not only have different contents, but also different forms. However, they share a common underlying feature in that they are organized interpretations of events. These interpretations will vary in complexity and will change in detail and structure across settings. They will also vary in their mode of transmission from everyday conversation to written, aural and visual forms.

Narrative psychology is particularly interested in the stories people tell themselves and others about their everyday experiences and those of others. In addition, it is interested in the shared narrative accounts of the families, communities and societies in which people grow up and which give shape to their lives and identities. The role of the narrative researcher is to explore the character of these different types of narrative, and how they connect with everyday social life.

Because we live in a world of narratives, researchers have many potential sources of data. The most popular source of research data is the interview but we can also look at stories conveyed on television and radio, in newspapers and books, in music and song, and in visual images. Such a wide range of sources can be confusing and for this reason we focus in this chapter on narratives obtained in interviews.

In looking at these narrative accounts we are interested in the character of the stories told, the language used, how it connects with particular experiences, how it can change, the way it is shared with others, and so on. The focus of our analysis will be dependent upon the research question.

Qualitative Research Methods in Mental Health and Psychotherapy: A Guide for Students and Practitioners, First Edition.
Edited by D. Harper and A.R. Thompson.
© 2012 John Wiley & Sons, Ltd. Published 2012 by John Wiley & Sons, Ltd.

Historical Origins and Influences

While interest in the character and role of narrative can be traced back to ancient times, it is only more recently that it has attracted substantial interest among psychologists. Here we will refer particularly to several important contributions in the 1980s.

In 1986, Mishler published his classic work on *Research Interviewing*. While formally this book was concerned with the collection and analysis of verbal data in interviews, throughout Mishler emphasized the importance of considering interviewee accounts as narratives or stories. In the appendix he provides an excellent summary of some of the key works that influenced his thinking on narrative. One of these was the historian White (1980) who noted: 'So natural is the impulse to narrate, so inevitable is the form of narrative for any report of the way things really happened, that narrativity could appear problematical only in a culture in which it was absent' (p. 5).

In the same year Sarbin published *Narrative Psychology: The storied nature of human conduct* (Sarbin, 1986). In this work he argued that whereas the machine metaphor underlay much of contemporary psychological theorizing, a more appropriate metaphor was that of narrative. He went on to argue that narrative was actually more than a metaphor for psychology but was a description of how people viewed the world.

Also in 1986, Bruner published *Actual Minds, Possible Worlds* in which he argued that there are two main forms of thinking – the paradigmatic and the narrative (Bruner, 1986). Whereas much psychological work was concerned with scientific thinking in everyday life, people organize their interpretations of the world in storied forms. The urge to develop a narrative account is particularly pronounced when the person experiences something different or exceptional.

Since these influential works were published there has been a steady stream of work which has explored ways of conducting narrative research, particularly within health psychology (e.g., Crossley, 1999; Murray, 1999).

Key Epistemological Assumptions

Narrative psychology is derived from the hermeneutic phenomenological tradition of Heideigger and Gadamer. In contrast to the more descriptive forms of phenomenology, hermeneutic phenomenology is concerned with how we interpret the world around us. Of particular importance is the French philosopher Ricoeur who argued that the meaning of the world is not transparent, but is instead mediated through the symbolic apparatus of culture. In Ricoeur's words: 'The referent of narration, namely human action, is never raw or immediate reality but an action which has been symbolized and resymbolized over and over again' (Ricoeur, 1991, p. 469).

We live in a world of constant change. The creation of narratives provides a sense of order and meaning to this change. While there may be sequences to certain events, humans interpret these sequences in different ways and provide different narrative accounts within which they place different emphases. They can also draw upon more established narratives to make sense of their world.

Narratives are also told in context. Thus, we are not telling stories in a vacuum but rather to another person. The context of storytelling is therefore important in understanding the particular shape of the narrative, especially when interpreting the narrative account obtained in an interview. Mishler (1986) referred explicitly to the power differential in the traditional interview. The challenge is for the narrative interviewer to reduce this power imbalance to encourage the narrator to expand upon their accounting. In some cases this can involve the researcher deliberately working to empower the participants through reflecting on the character of their narrative account (see below). When the researcher takes time to listen they will often find that the narrator will enthusiastically take advantage of the opportunity to tell their stories in great detail.

Narrative is also of central importance in understanding identity. It is through telling stories to ourselves and to others that we define ourselves. Narrative provides continuity in our sense of self. Ricoeur identified the plot as the central structure of any narrative and the process of emplotment as central to narrative making; it is the 'synthesis of heterogenous elements' (Ricoeur, 1991, p. 426). In the same way, in emplotting one's life story, one defines one's identity. This argument was taken up in developmental psychology by McAdams who argued that 'the problem of identity is the problem of arriving at a life story that makes sense – provides unity and purpose – within a sociohistorical matrix that embodies a much larger story' (McAdams, 1988, p. 18). Thus, our identity and our world are defined in terms of stories within stories.

Types of Research Questions

Contemporary interest in narrative within the health arena focuses on the 'stories' that patients/clients tell about their experiences of having particular health problems. Adopting a phenomenological perspective the narrative researcher can begin with a broad question about the experience of living with a health problem. Thus, the researcher might adopt a life history approach in encouraging the participant to narrate their biographical experiences, thereby locating the illness experience within a broader life course perspective. In interpreting this account the researcher is interested in how the narrative is structured, how the language is used and the connection with other experiences. For example, the researcher might be interested in the experience of living with disability. Murray (2007) conducted biographical interviews with men who had suffered serious occupational injury leading to them being unable to work full time. In interpreting these narrative accounts Murray connected their experience of disability with their other life experiences as manual workers, as husbands and as community members. The researcher might also be interested in certain aspects of participants' encounters with a health or social agency. Again, in the example above, Murray (2007) considered how the workers viewed the government agency concerned with providing financial support for those on long-term disability. A particular source of frustration expressed by the men was the questioning of their accounts by the agency. In interpreting these narratives an important issue was how the men defined themselves as responsible and active agents. They were angry at the system because of the perceived challenge to their identity. However, this challenge could not be rebutted by a return to work so instead they became entwined in a conflict with the agency to justify their claim to disability.

Sorts of Data

The primary sources of data are interview transcripts. Interviews can focus on particular life events or on the whole life history of the interviewees. While the focus may be on a particular health issue there is the opportunity to contextualize this within their broader life history and social context. Thus, the researcher could encourage the participant to talk about their encounters with a particular health professional. In this case the researcher would prompt the participants to provide as much detail as possible about their actual encounters. The researcher could also obtain detail on other life experiences of the individuals and their encounters with other health services.

Subsequently, these interviews would be transcribed. The most common form of transcription is to include the words of both the interviewer and the participant, to number the transcribed lines, and to indicate paralinguistics such as emphases or pauses.

Some researchers will deliberately reformat the raw transcript into other linguistic forms. For example, Gee (1991) (see Chapter 9) has suggested looking at the poetic form that underlies some narrative accounts. Here, the researcher is particularly interested in the rhythm of the narrative account and the use of metaphor.

Outputs such as diaries may carry the benefit of being able to see the proportionate influence that mental ill health can have on daily life. They provide an opportunity to clearly connect events with particular time periods and contexts, and the changing positions that individuals assume. They can also give insight into the extent to which health and illness may feature in someone's account, thereby providing more information on how the content of distress features, and how mental health difficulties occur across time, rather than at one particular isolated moment.

Involvement of Research Participants

Providing participants with the opportunity to describe their experiences in detail can be immensely invigorating for them. Thus, while the narrative interview is not formally a therapy session it can be therapeutic. Indeed, Mishler (1986) emphasized this point: 'The effort to empower respondents and the study of their responses as narratives are closely interlinked. They are connected through the assumption ... that one of the significant ways through which individuals make sense of and give meaning to their experiences is to organize them in a narrative form' (p. 118).

He continued: 'Through their narratives people may be moved beyond the text to the possibilities of action. That is, to be empowered is not only to speak in one's own voice and to tell one's own story, but to apply the understanding arrived at to action in accord with one's own interests' (Mishler, 1986, p. 119).

Much of narrative research does not have that process as its primary goal. Rather, the usual intention is to collect the narrative accounts and then to subject these accounts to analysis. However, in some projects the participants are involved individually or collectively in exploring the character of their narratives and their connections with everyday life. For example, Weingarten actively considered the process of making sense of her own narratives about her experience of breast cancer. She found that Gergen's (1994) narrative classification scheme offered her a means of 'resisting the diminishment of personhood that Western cultural ideas about fitness, accomplishment success, individualism, and progress would have me feel' (see http://www.dulwichcentre.com.au/illness-narratives.html). With the researcher the narrator can consider the emphasis placed on certain issues, the actual language and metaphors used, and the overall structure of the narrative as possibly being fractured or coherent. However, the clinical researcher needs to be sensitive to the ethical issues involved in the different roles that they can have as both a clinician and as a researcher (see Chapter 3). A group of participants can share their stories and then reflect upon them together. This then can become a form of action research as the participants identify shared experiences (e.g., of their frustration with certain aspects of health care), identifying sources of distress (e.g., access to care) and can also consider ways of tackling these. In a study of a support group for people with chronic fatigue syndrome, Bulow (2004) described the centrality of shared narrative making in the group. It was through this process that the participants developed a mutual understanding of their own illness experiences.

This collaborative process of narrative making can also become part of a participatory research project. For example, in a study of homeless women (Washington & Moxley, 2008) the researchers initially collected narratives from the women of their experiences. Together they developed an exhibition which highlighted the challenges they experienced. This process of narrative sharing thus becomes a means of empowerment, and also potentially leads to forms of social action and change. Another example is the work of Schneider (2010) who worked with a group of people with schizophrenia to create a performance and a graphic novel about their experiences (http://callhome.ucalgary.ca/performances/index.html).

Details of Using Method

Narrative analysis can provide a way of connecting everyday concerns that are not always related to illness but are inextricably linked to it. These issues can include aspects of embodiment, biography, living space and personal relationships. There are certain characteristics of narratives about which we must be aware to examine them successfully. A theme, plot, structure, characters, a narrator, a setting, time and causality are components that help us to manage our understanding of individual and institutional/collective narratives. It is important to note, however, that an analysis of all these components is not necessarily required – as with other qualitative analytic strategies, it is acceptable to focus on fewer aspects, or even just one. Here we will consider some of these aspects.

Structure

One of the earliest documented methods of narrative analysis is the structured approach of Labov and Waletsky (1967), which proposed a systematic way of compartmentalizing a narrative. This involves seeking particular aspects of a story, including the *orientation, complicating action* and *evaluation*. At the most simplified level, the orientation is the 'scene-setting' of a particular narrative (stating where or when a situation occurred). The complicating action is the essence of the story and the reason for it being told, and the evaluation is the point at which the story is concluded and summarized. There are other stages that fall in between these structural parts, but overall this illustrates how a story can be partitioned for lateral analysis across several cases.

The following example is taken from a study of how young people adjust to inflammatory bowel disease (Sargeant *et al.* 2005). The interview extract on the left below describes a hospital visit, in which the participant and his consultant were discussing treatment options, and his wish to minimize anxiety for his parents. The coding on the right breaks down the extract in terms of how it might appear within a Labovian structure.

This was just before Christmas, a couple of days before and I went home and my mum was like, well, how was it at the hospital? And I was like yes, fine. And she went like is there any new information or stuff? And I was like no, no, they're just going to stick on with the old stuff [*treatment regime*]. Because she was – her and my dad were going away on holiday on Boxing Day and if I'd gone to my mum oh no, I've got to have an operation, she'd be like oh, I'm not going then, not going on holiday [. . .] I was like hmm, I've got to – got to keep schtum about this one because I knew she'd react and she'd try and cancel the holiday. So then like she (inaudible) oh, we're fine to go and things like that, and things escalate don't they? So I just thought best keep it under wraps, let Christmas pass.	ORIENTATION: the particpant begins by providing context of who, when and where

ABSTRACT: here it emerges what the story is about

The COMPLICATING ACTION is the revelation of concealment of events

The participant's EVALUATION gives the reason for his actions

RESULT: the character (participant's mother) asserts that they can travel

CODA: the participant summarizes, and brings the context back to the start – Christmas |

This veers more towards simple description in breaking down the story in this way, and can sometimes be at the expense of other interpretative elements of a narrative. However, it is a useful way to begin a narrative analysis, especially as such accounts may be presented by people in a clinical therapeutic setting. In terms of beginning to examine narratives, a structured approach can be a beginning towards understanding narratives as sequential processes. It can also help to identify further elements, such as coherence.

Coherence

One theoretical model that focuses on psychological well-being defines narrative coherence by using four interrelated features: orientation, structure, affect and integration (Baerger & McAdams, 1999). Orientation provides the reader/audience with the background information necessary to tell the story. Structure relates to the temporal ordering of a narrative and affect refers to the emotional components.

The final aspect, integration, is described as 'the required and sustained effort on the part of the life story narrator to synthesize the pieces of a life into a story' (Baerger & McAdams, 1999, p. 78). The study involved 50 adults completing various life satisfaction scales, then being asked to describe specific events (e.g., a nadir experience, a turning point scene, an adolescent experience). These were then coded using the four indices mentioned above, using a Likert scale, 1 being 'very low' to 7 being 'very high'. Participants were given scores for each life story episode and an overall coherence score. The central argument was that life story coherence is measurable and related to psychological well-being, with the principal assertion that a good life story exhibits coherence that extends beyond temporal or sequential ordering.

It is also worth pointing out *different* types of coherence. Habermas and Bluck (2002) characterize narrative by four types of coherence: temporal, thematic, casual and biographical. The authors charted this by using these four types as pivots for their argument, and stated that the tools for constructing a life story develop in adolescence. However, they did not separate the life story framework from other research areas, such as coping, therapeutic processes and the organization of autobiographical memory. While a life story may not present all-inclusive coherence, it still offers resources that clearly present themselves for further scrutiny, as aspects of narrative coherence are fragmented rather than whole entities within accounts.

Emplotment

A concept related to that of coherence is emplotment. This term was introduced by Ricoeur and describes the process of bringing material together to create a narrative. Thus, the plot provides not just coherence but a sense of direction to the narrative. This was also explored by Mattingly (1998) who examined the relationships between storytelling and improvement in health status based on her observations of occupational therapists working with elderly infirm patients. The patients' respective illnesses are unspecified, but Mattingly describes therapists' concentrations on getting the patients to move their limbs with a clinical aim of improving coordination, while ignoring their sudden reminiscences of life events.

These observations illustrate the importance of personal stories and also reveal the emerging conflicts between treatment agendas and patient needs. This also points to the omissions that can arise in clinical practice in terms of accounting for the events in life that would not otherwise warrant attention if studying aspects of health and illness. Overall, Mattingly's recommendation was for an observer/analyst to encourage a service user to plot their experiences, rather than to focus specifically on the problem to be solved, which is very much the premise of narrative therapy (White & Epston, 1990). Such recommendations are easily transposed into mental health with the emphasis upon divergence from the condition being treated and instead encouraging the production of narratives that can be related to the illness in question. The context in which Mattingly situates emplotment strategies here relates specifically to how a therapist/health professional can facilitate a service user's narration, therefore paying particular attention to using the narrative as a practitioner and active interviewer, as well as an analyst of talk and text.

Positioning

When people produce narratives their 'plots' can change over time, and so too can their *positions*. 'Positioning' is a term that features in Chapter 11 and the references listed there will assist in narrative analysis. In addition to the material there, Bamberg (2004) offers a positioning theory that also helps in examining narrative accounts and suggests two forces that can operate within stories. These forces are simplified as person-to-world and world-to-person directions in narrative accounts. Bamberg defined the former as a 'subject being determined by the outside', mainly social and biological forces, and the latter being 'the unitary subject as ground'. Consider the following extract, taken from an audio diary sequence from a young person with a diagnosis of Crohn's disease (Sargeant *et al.*, 2009):

> Sorry I'm only doing this weekly but school so mad and I haven't got much time at the moment. I prefer it on a weekly basis – um, what was I going to say about this week? Pretty much the same as last week really. Homework starting to settle down now I'm getting back into a rhythm, it's good in that respect – it's a calm week. My Crohn's is still playing up a bit, and um been having the cramps and stuff, been having to go to matron in lessons cos I just can't stand it anymore and I have to have a hot water bottle. The medications – putting me back on, they're taking me off diclofenac [*medication*], then they put me back on, then there are different tablets, very confusing. In a few weeks when it's settled down I'll put a medication entry in explaining all that, but it's just too complicated at the moment [...]

> Oh, did you know, I'm in a band? That's what I was going to tell you. Some of my friends are in a boy band, so we decided to do ours I think I've already mentioned Blank Page [*name of a band*], but that sounds really cheesy. We decided not to do that cos that was just a bit – that was just to annoy the boys. But anyway, my friend is having guitar lessons. They've put me on drums cos I've got a drum set up in my room, such a laugh as none of us know quite what we're doing really. On the practices – if you can call them practices really it's just gossiping, just a bit weird really.

This is a good example of changing positions. It begins with the participant trying to establish a routine in her busy schoolwork schedule, in which she is the driver of the narrative: the person-to-world position. By the fourth line, she reveals that her illness has caused disruption to that routine. This could be interpreted as a change in positioning direction – a shift to a 'world-to-person' view, as shown through the lines 'They're taking me off diclofenac' and 'Mum tells me what tablets to take'. The shift is, perhaps, a relinquishing of control. Finally, the position reverts to a person-to-world perspective, wherein the participant speaks about activities she controls. Therefore the key outcome of conducting a narrative analysis from this theoretical perspective is the understanding that position shifts can occur within the same account, as well as between different ones.

Bamberg's approach lends itself to the examination of mental health/illness narratives. A further simplification of this would be to examine data to see how and where illness features over time. Sargeant *et al.* (2009) proposed the following definitions:

- *Illness absent:* an account in which illnesses and related matters are unmentioned, such as a description of an ordinary activity, or something exceptional such as attending a concert.
- *Illness embedded:* an account that begins as a narrative unrelated to illness, but illness-related concerns emerge during the course of the account. An example might include a description of an event, within which a 'cue' renders an inclusion of an illness-related content that is not the driving force of the narrative.
- *Illness directed:* an account explicitly about illness. An example might include a service user account of a mental health review meeting in which the health issues are clearly governing the narrative, rather than occurring within it as might be seen with an 'embedded' illness narrative.

By using this simplified definition, the extract above can be perhaps categorized as a 'disease embedded' account, in which the participant begins her account with unrelated activities, and then moves through to speaking of her illness, then moving again to distance herself from it with her revelation of non-diseased related activity.

Where to start?

Deciding which narrative aspect to focus upon depends on the research question and the character of the data. An initial analysis of any account may look for information on a thematic basis, especially if much of the narrative is verbalized and not in textual format. A further development may be to elicit a written narrative (e.g., suggesting that a person produce a written diary of events relevant to them that are part of a therapeutic process). From this a more detailed level of analysis may be undertaken, such as identifying the way in which a narrative is 'resolved' from a Labovian perspective.

Quality Issues

In collecting narrative accounts similar quality issues arise as for other forms of qualitative research. There is a need for care in collecting, transcribing and coding the interview data which is the common source of material. In collecting accounts it is important to provide sufficient opportunity for the interviewee to develop their narratives. This requires time and possibly repeated meetings with the interviewee. Caution should be exercised in collecting accounts of crises, the detail of which can be emotionally difficult for both the narrator and the researcher. Even details of more mundane events can encourage recollection of more traumatic events.

In coding the narrative accounts the emphasis is on seeing the whole of the account rather than rushing to break it up into parts. The advice of Mishler (1986) to avoid the interruptions typical of traditional researchers remains relevant: 'interviewers interrupt respondents' answers and thereby suppress expression of their stories; when they appear, stories go unrecorded because they are viewed as irrelevant to the specific aims of specific questions; and stories that make it through these barriers are discarded at stages of coding and analysis (Mishler, 1986, p. 106).

While the researcher can consider the various parts of the narrative account and the use of metaphors and particular expressions, they should not lose sight of its overall structure and how it is oriented.

'Evidence' and Policy

There is much contemporary debate about the 'impact' of research. Narrative research is particularly valuable because of its potential to actively engage participants in the research process and in the interpretation and dissemination of the research. Thus, the participant can be encouraged through the research to reflect upon the structure of the narrative and how this connects with their everyday lives. Narrative accounts are also immensely powerful in convincing people of the legitimacy of a particular argument. For example, in the study of deliberative democracy in the health service, Davies *et al.* (2006) found that lay members of the citizen councils were often bored by more abstract material and deliberately requested more personalized details from the expert witnesses. The researchers concluded that although the narrative style of speech was formally discouraged it was held in higher esteem by the lay members. The hearing of narrative accounts provided certain legitimacy to more abstract formulations.

Within what has become known as participatory policy research there have been deliberate attempts to integrate narrative research. For example, Orsini and Scala (2006) argue that narrative research can be a means of 'bringing the patient back in' to health care which has become dominated by the tenets of evidence-based medicine. In particular, they illustrate how narrative approaches can draw attention to newly emerging illnesses as well as often to ignored chronic illnesses.

There have been attempts to formalize how to introduce narrative analysis into the policy process. Hampton (2004) details how to identify dominant and hidden or counter narratives within any policy debate. It is through this process that issues of social injustice can be exposed and new narratives developed.

Recent Developments

There are increasing numbers of studies of narrative. On the one hand, we can point to the popularity of first person accounts of particular mental health problems by both professionals (e.g., Ron Bassman's account of his personal experience of schizophrenia; http://ronaldbassman.com/) and by non-professionals (e.g., Bassett & Stickley, 2010). The widespread interest in these popular accounts is a cultural phenomenon which may reflect the increasing challenge to more scientific approaches to health and the greater participation of patients/clients in health care decision making. These public stories can be used in an advocacy role and also as a means of sharing experiences (see also on-line discussion groups) as well as part of professional development. Indeed, there are increasing examples of narrative accounts being used to promote discussion about particular illness experiences (e.g., http://www.storyworksglam.co.uk). This is coupled with the growth of interest in digital storytelling which is a way of combining recorded voice, still and moving images, and various sounds (see http://www.storycenter.org).

This use of narrative accounts to promote change overlaps with the growth of narrative therapy. While there has been much development in explicating this method it is sufficient here to note that the telling and sharing of stories of illness experiences can be therapeutic for the narrator. This idea has been taken up by a number of psychologists (e.g., Mathieson & Stam, 1996) to explore the 'biographical work' engaged in by (ex) patients in integrating the illness experience into their larger narrative identities. For example, Ville (2005) detailed the character of the biographical work carried out by people who had become paraplegic. Initially, they were concerned with coming to terms with their impairment but later biographical work involved them considering employment opportunities. This raises the questions about the role of the health researcher as both a clinician and as a researcher. While in the research setting the storytelling may be therapeutic to the teller it should not be considered as a formal therapy session. The challenge is for the clinician-researcher to remain aware of the particular ethical issues of the two roles (see Chapter 3).

In their study of psychiatric consumer/survivors, Nelson et al. (2001) detail the different personal narrative accounts. Reviewing these accounts, Nelson et al. highlight the movement from powerlessness to feelings of control which were facilitated by community mental health programmes. This illustrated Rappaport's (1995) argument that individual change is facilitated by a supportive context that challenges the dominant negative social narrative of mental illness.

A final example of the use of narrative theory as the framework for a community intervention is the work by Murray and Crummett (2010) on older people's perceptions of their disadvantaged neighbourhood. They found that the older people characterized their neighbourhood in terms of a narrative of decline leading to feelings of fatalism. Through participation in a community arts project, the older residents began to challenge that narrative through the process of social action.

These studies illustrate how research using narrative as a framework has moved from investigating individual narrative accounts of human distress to more societal narratives of change and resistance. Recently, Selbin (2010) has used narrative as an integrative framework for understanding revolution and rebellion. It is through the sharing of stories of transformation that people can begin to believe in the possibility of change and to take action to achieve such change whether it is at the local level or at a broader level.

References

Baerger, D.R. & McAdams, D. (1999). Life story coherence and its relation to psychological well-being. *Narrative Inquiry, 9*, 69–96.

Bamberg, M. (2004). Positioning with Davie Hogan; stories, tellings and identities. In C. Lightfoot & C. Daiute (Eds.) *Narrative analysis: Studying the development of individuals in society* (pp. 133–157). London: Sage.

Bassett, T. & Stickley, T. (Eds.) (2010). *Voices of experience: Narratives of mental health survivors.* London: Wiley-Blackwell.

Bruner, J. (1986). *Actual minds, possible worlds.* Cambridge, MA: Harvard University Press.

Bulow, P.H. (2004). Sharing experiences of contested illness by storytelling. *Discourse and Society, 15*, 33–53.

Crossley, M.L. (1999). *Introducing narrative psychology: Self, trauma and the construction of meaning.* Buckingham, Open University Press.

Davies, C., Wetherell, M. & Barnett, E. (2006). *Citizens at the centre: Deliberative participation in healthcare decisions.* Bristol: Policy Press.

Gee, J.P. (1991). A linguistic approach to narrative. *Journal of Narrative and Life History/Narrative Inquiry, 1*, 15–39.

Gergen, K. (1994). *Realities and relationships: Soundings in social construction.* Cambridge, MA: Harvard University Press.

Habermas, T. & Bluck, S. (2002). Getting a life: The emergence of the life story in adolescence. *Psychological Bulletin, 126*, 748–769.

Hampton, G. (2004). Enhancing public participation through narrative analysis. *Policy Sciences, 37*, 261–276.

Labov, W. & Waletsky, J. (1967). Narrative analysis: Oral versions of personal experience. In J. Helm (Ed.) *Essays on the verbal and visual arts* (pp. 12–44). Seattle: University of Washington Press.

Mathieson, C. & Stam, H.J. (1995). Renegotiating identity: cancer narratives. *Sociology of Health and Illness, 17*, 283–306.

Mattingly, C. (1998). *Healing dramas and clinical plots.* Los Angeles, CA: University of California Press.

McAdams, D. (1988). *Power, intimacy and the life story: Personological inquiries into identity.* New York: Guilford Press.

Mishler, E.G. (1986). *Research interviewing: Context and narrative.* Cambridge, MA: Harvard University Press.

Murray, M. (1999). The storied nature of health and illness. In M. Murray & K. Chamberlain (Eds.) *Qualitative health psychology: Theories and methods* (pp. 47–63). London: Sage.

Murray, M. (2007). 'It's in the blood and you're not going to change it': Fish harvesters' narrative accounts of injuries and disability. *WORK, 28*, 165–174.

Murray, M. & Crummett, A. (2010). 'I don't think they knew we could do these sorts of things': Social representations of community and participation in community arts by older people. *Journal of Health Psychology, 15*, 777–785.

Nelson, G., Lord, J. & Ochocka, J. (2001). Empowerment and mental health in community: Narratives of psychiatric consumer/survivors. *Journal of Community and Applied Social Psychology, 11*, 125–142.

Orsini, M. & Scala, F. (2006). Every virus tells a story: Toward a narrative centered approach to health policy. *Policy and Society, 25*, 109–130.

Rappaport, J. (1995). Empowerment meets narrative: Listening to stories and creating settings. *American Journal of Community Psychology, 23*, 795–807.

Ricoeur, P. (1981). The creativity of language. In M.J. Valdes (Ed.) (1991). *A Ricoeur reader: Reflection and imagination* (pp. 461–481). Toronto: University of Toronto Press.

Ricoeur, P. (1987). Life in search of a narrator. In M.J. Valdes (Ed.) (1991). *A Ricoeur reader: Reflection and imagination* (pp. 425–437). Toronto: University of Toronto Press.

Sarbin, T. (Ed.) (1986). *Narrative psychology: The storied nature of human conduct.* New York: Praeger.

Sargeant, S., Gross, H. & Middleton, D.J. (2005). Public conveniences, private matters: Retrospective narration of adolescent daily life with inflammatory bowel disease. In N. Kelly, C. Horrocks, K. Milnes, B. Roberts & D. Robinson (Eds.) *Narrative, memory and everyday life* (pp. 143–151). Huddersfield: University of Huddersfield Press.

Sargeant, S., Gross, H. & Middleton, D. (2009). Two worlds, one life: Narrative spaces of identity between health and illness. In D. Robinson, C. Horrocks, N. Kelly & B. Roberts (Eds.) *Narrative, memory and identity* (pp. 95–103). Huddersfield: University of Huddersfield Press.

Schneider, B. (2010). *Hearing (our) voices: Participatory research in mental health.* Toronto: University of Toronto Press.

Selbin, E. (2010). *Revolution, rebellion, resistance: The power of story.* London: Zed Books.

Ville, I. (2005). Biographical work and returning to employment following a spinal cord injury. *Sociology of Health and Illness, 27*, 324–350.

Washington, O.G.M. & Moxley, D.P. (2008). Telling my story: From narrative to exhibit in illuminating the lived experience of homelessness among older African American women. *Journal of Health Psychology, 13*, 154–165.

White, H. (1980). The value of narrativity in the representations of reality. *Critical Inquiry, 7*, 5–27.

White, M. & Epston, D. (1990). *Narrative means to therapeutic ends.* New York: W.W. Norton.

Further reading and useful website

Bamberg, M. (Ed.) (2007). *Narrative: State of the art.* Amsterdam: John Benjamins. [An excellent selection of articles on narrative]

http://dulwichcentre.com.au/ [An expanding online resource of narrative practice and research]

Laszlo, J. (2008). *The science of stories: An introduction to narrative psychology.* London: Routledge. [An overview of current approaches to narrative psychology]

13

Ethnomethodology/Conversation Analysis

Mark Rapley

Ethnomethodology is working out some very preposterous problems. (Garfinkel, 2002, p. 91)

[D]etailed study of small phenomena may give an enormous understanding of the way humans do things and the kinds of objects they use to construct and order their affairs. (Sacks, 1984, p. 24)

Ethnomethodology/Conversation Analysis

As may be surmised from the quotes above, Ethnomethodology/Conversation Analysis (EM/CA) has no recognizable method, qua 'method'. There are no formalized procedures, 39 steps or arcane methodological practices. This is not to say that there is not an orderly way to go about doing this sort of work (see Box 13.1 for tenHave's suggested process; for a more detailed discussion see tenHave, 2001, 2007), but the trick is to get interested in what you have got. That is to say: 'we sit down with a piece of data, make a bunch of observations, and see where they will go' (Sacks, 1984, p. 27). What best characterizes EM/CA – despite its diversity and heterogeneity (and sometimes vitriolic internal disagreements: Carlin, 2010; Schegloff, 2007a,b) – is then not a set of *methods*, but rather an *analytic mentality* (Schenkein, 1978), or 'a shared orientation to an extant, achieved orderliness in everyday activities and a commitment to discovering organizational features of direct interaction' (Maynard & Clayman, 1991, p. 385).

EM/CA seeks to uncover 'seen but unnoticed' aspects of the doing of everyday life: 'to discover the things that persons in particular situations *do*, the methods *they* use, to create the patterned orderliness of social life' (Garfinkel, 2002, p. 6). The range of the

Qualitative Research Methods in Mental Health and Psychotherapy: A Guide for Students and Practitioners, First Edition.
Edited by D. Harper and A.R. Thompson.
© 2012 John Wiley & Sons, Ltd. Published 2012 by John Wiley & Sons, Ltd.

Box 13.1 A General Outline for Conversation Analysis Research Projects

1. Make complete and detailed transcriptions of the recordings

Making detailed transcriptions first, and working with simplified versions for specific purposes later, is recommended because it makes these details available for unforeseen and unforeseeable analytic benefits

2. A general strategy for data exploration

2.1   Starting with an arbitrarily or purposively selected part of the transcribed data, work through the transcript in terms of a restricted set of analytically distinguished, but interlocking, 'organizations'

2.2   For this purpose the following four are helpful: turn-taking organization; sequence organization; repair organization; organization of turn-design. This 'work through' involves a turn-by-turn consideration of the data in terms of practices relevant to these essential organizations, such as taking a turn in a specific way, initiating a sequence, foregoing taking up an issue, and so on. In other words, the task is to *specify practice/action couplings* as these are available in the data, where the actions are as far as possible formulated in terms of the four organizations

2.3   On the basis of this process, try to *formulate some general observations, statements, or rules that tentatively summarize what has been seen.* When a particular interest or phenomenon has emerged, focus on it, but keep it in context in terms of these four organizations

3. A general strategy for data elaboration

Try to use a substantial corpus of data which, while relevant for the purpose at hand, has not been pre-selected with any particular notion, expectation or hypothesis in mind. Except for projects that are targeted at phenomena that have a principled structural 'place' within the temporal development of an encounter, or established interactional role, try to work with complete, start-to-finish recordings of the phenomena/events to be investigated

3.1   Start with a single case analysis, following the suggestions for analytic exploration, resulting in an *analytic summary*

3.2   After this, select another piece of data, and work through that piece of data again in terms of the four organizations. Mark the observations you make in terms of their fit with the tentative summary. Revise the summary as required to accommodate both old and the new data. Repeat this with subsequent parts of the data until you have processed the complete corpus

(Continued)

Box 13.1 (*Cont'd*)

3.3   Identify any *deviant* instances in the data and explicate their relationship with otherwise regular patterns observed

3.4   Rework the summary as it has been revised in terms of its comprehensiveness of data coverage. You may need to distinguish types of conversational devices, alternative solution to interactional troubles, and so on

3.5   Construct a *summary formulation* that covers the general findings, the variation of types, and deviant cases

—Adapted from tenHave (2010), with permission.

work is vast, encompassing such topics as how people do waiting for a bus (Sharrock, 1995); doing psychotherapy (Peräkylä *et al.*, 2008); teenagers categorizing themselves in therapy sessions (Sacks, 1992); being a schizophrenic or a person with an intellectual disability (Rapley, 2004; Wise & Rapley, 2009); diagnosing attention deficit hyperactivity disorder (ADHD; McHoul & Rapley, 2005); calling suicide helplines (Sacks, 1992); to managing football clubs (Rapley & McHoul, 2002).

CA is a branching out from Sacks' elaboration of Garfinkel's original work in ethnomethodology (McHoul, 2008). CA – and related approaches such as Membership Categorization Analysis (MCA; Hester & Eglin, 1997) – are not separate fields but rather EM, CA and MCA, and more recent developments such as discursive psychology (Edwards, 1995; Edwards & Potter, 1992; McHoul & Rapley, 2000) adopt different analytic emphases.

This approach is grounded in looking *outwards* into the world; it is not that EM/CA has nothing to say about matters such as cognition (Potter, 2006; teMolder & Potter, 2005) or specific psychological issues such as 'theory of mind' (Leudar & Costall, 2009), but that the approach is, essentially, interested in the viewable, verifiable and accountable rather than the invisible, hypothetical and theoretical.

Historical Origins

EM/CA derives from the sociological work of Garfinkel (1967, 2002) who invented the term 'ethnomethodology', which in turn influenced Sacks and colleagues who developed what is known as CA. Garfinkel drew on work in 'structural' (or 'archetectonic'; Heritage, 1984, p. 33) sociology (particularly Weber, Durkheim and Parsons); the philosophy of Heidegger and Wittgenstein, and the phenomenology of Schütz. EM/CA offers a radical counter to traditional sociology, and continues to be at odds with mainstream positivist sociology and more recent post-modern/post-structuralist variants.

Equally, whilst not focusing directly on psychological matters, EM/CA offers a challenge to individualistic psychology (Coulter, 1979; McHoul & Rapley, 2000; Potter, 2006). Following Goffman's studies of the 'interaction order', what Garfinkel formulated in EM, and Sacks elaborated in CA, was an insistence on paying close attention to the witnessable: not speculating about a mysterious interiority or theorizing 'variables' such as 'gender' or 'class' except where made relevant by members in interaction.

Key Epistemological Assumptions

Forms of life are always forms of life forming.

Realities are always realities becoming. (Mehan & Wood, 1975, p. 32)

EM/CA is informed by a small number of epistemological assumptions but does not sit easily on a 'realism–relativism continuum': it is 'realist' in the sense that it deals in 'realities' or 'social facts' (Garfinkel, 2002), and grounds its claims in empirical data, but is 'relativist' in that the *indexicality* of action – the insistence that 'realities are always realities becoming' – is central. Hence, what a given utterance is to be understood as, or what a specific social action accomplishes, are not *fixed* 'facts', but rather (co-)constructed in their haecceity, in and for their moment of use, within ongoing orderly streams of (inter)action. Indeed, EM/CA is extraordinarily attentive to how the 'facticity' of social facts is actually achieved (Lynch & Bogen, 1996; Rapley, 1998).

The kinds of claims made by EM/CA are not, however, probabilistic or normative in the *statistical* sense: EM/CA describes the *regularly observable* and argues that the details of phenomena observed (be they conversations, bus queues or psychotherapy) are massively reproducible. This is not to claim that *all* conversational openings, bus queues or psychotherapy sessions do, or must, occur in a standardized fashion – what is known as 'deviant case analysis', the detailed study of apparently disconfirmatory findings, is an important verification procedure in EM/CA for interrogating the 'truth status' of observations – but to say that it is a demonstrably pervasive feature of human sociality that things routinely happen in an orderly, and ordered, fashion.

Ethnomethodological indifference

EM/CA adopts a stance of *ethnomethodological indifference* (Garfinkel & Sacks, 1970) – suspending disciplinary knowledge (be it sociological or psychological) as historically situated understandings themselves amenable to analysis. So, rather than assuming, a priori, that certain forms of talk (e.g., 'word salad') index 'schizophrenia', EM/CA examines *how* the existence of such things-in-the-world as 'schizophrenia' are brought off in, by, and through – for example – interactions with professionals. That is, EM/CA shows the operation, in operation, of the interactional practices via which 'schizophrenia' is 'talked into being' *as such* (Heritage, 1984, p. 290).

Rejection of cultural dopism

EM/CA has a fundamental respect for the practical knowledge of ordinary members (of society). Sacks makes this point clearly:

> There's a place in Freud where he says, 'with regard to matters of chemistry or physics or things like that, laymen would not venture an opinion. With regard to psychology it's quite different; anybody feels free to make psychological remarks'. And part of the business he thought he was engaged in was changing that around . . . [S]o that laymen would know that they don't know anything about it and that there are people who do, so that they would eventually stop making psychological remarks (Sacks, 1992, p. 217).

EM/CA suggests that ordinary people are treated by sociology and psychology as 'cultural dopes' (Garfinkel, 1984, p. 68): driven by social – or intra-psychic – forces of which they are unaware, and which require expert explanation (McHoul & Rapley, 2003). Unlike mainstream social science, EM/CA adopts a non-ironic stance towards the (accounting) practices of members. What this means is that EM/CA accepts that members' procedural knowledge may be tacit, but as part of the very cultural machinery that EM/CA seeks to understand, the (accounting) practices of members cannot simply be dismissed; rather, they are available for – and amenable to – analysis. The suspicion EM/CA has of the formalized theorizing of the social sciences is not only reflected in the insistence on taking the routine practices of ordinary life – and members' common sense mundane reasoning – seriously, but also in an epistemological commitment to the notion of 'order at all points' and, in consequence, a very different approach to 'sampling' to that of both quantitative social science and qualitative approaches such as Interpretative Phenomenological Analysis (IPA) and Grounded Theory which specify sampling quanta in an aspiration to representativeness.

'Order at all points'

EM/CA offers a radically different perspective on the representativeness of data, and the generalizability of its claims. This perspective is grounded in a view of human conduct quite dissimilar to the world view inherited from the physical sciences. As Sacks notes, the 'detailed study of small phenomena may give an enormous understanding' of much 'larger' social and cultural matters.

Schegloff describes the 'standard' position in the social sciences, and outlines the EM/CA position:

> [Sampling] depends on the sort of order one takes it that the social world exhibits. An alternative to the possibility that order manifests itself at an aggregate level and is statistical in character is . . . the 'order at all points' view. This view understands order not to be present only at aggregate levels and therefore subject to an overall differential distribution, but to *be present in detail on a case by case, environment by environment basis*. A culture is not then to be found only by aggregating all of its venues; it is substantially present in each (Schegloff in Sacks, 1992, p. xlvi).

'Traditional' statistical models of research then cannot but miss much of the essentially social/cultural grounds of human action (Rapley *et al.*, 2003). EM/CA suggests that a detailed examination of even the tiniest fragments of the social order reveals important properties of the whole. On this basis, EM/CA makes general claims about the ordering of social life, and by virtue of its assumption of order at all points, regards the study of few, or even single, instances as providing a sufficient basis for this.

The material reality of the social order: haecceity and indexicality

EM/CA is insistent upon the concrete material reality of the social order. But this is no naïve realism. Rather, EM/CA may be described (loosely) as 'constructionist': at the core of its epistemological position are the notions of *haecceity* and *indexicality*.

EM/CA regards the social order as a *self-generating* social order – in which the recognizable structures of the everyday are continuously and collaboratively brought into being *in their haecceity* (their uniqueness as what they are) – via the 'conversational and other methodic practices whereby members of society assemble social actions and the circumstances in which they are embedded' (Maynard & Clayman, 2003, p. 195). These actions are *indexical;* that is, their moment-of-use makes them what they are. Thus, a psychotherapy session, although sharing semantic (meaning) and prosodic (patterns of metre) structures with ordinary conversation is, recognizably, *not* 'an ordinary conversation'. Rather 'psychotherapy' is co-produced, as 'Psychotherapy', by the methodic, collaborative, deployment of *specifically patterned* conversational practices to produce interlocutors – in and for the moment – as PATIENT + THERAPIST not FRIEND + FRIEND.

The ongoing co-production of the social order – and persons such as 'therapists' and 'patients' within it – relies upon the *indexicality* of conduct, and of utterances. That is to say (cf. Wittgenstein, 1953) all forms of conduct – including utterances – are dependent for their meaning on the *occasion of their use*, or, as Wittgenstein says: 'our talk gets its meaning from the rest of our proceedings' (Wittgenstein, 1975, ¶ 229). It is from the fine-grained attention to the details of use that EM/CA derives its analytic power, and its ability to make persuasive observations by virtue of its refusal to stray from the data. EM/CA's 'empiricism is [then] that of the art critic who cites the pigments and brush strokes of the paintings he interprets' (Moerman, 1988; xiii).

The documentary method of interpretation

In accomplishing such an interpretation EM/CA relies on *witnessable* data. Garfinkel (1967) suggests that the *documentary method of interpretation* entails treating observables 'as pointing towards', or being a 'documentation of', underlying patterned-ness in social action. Like historians employing the 'documentary record' to reconstruct and – literally – to document otherwise anecdotal, interested or partial accounts, for EM/CA 'documents' serve to display patterns. Crucially, while these documents are interpreted on the basis of the assumption of underlying patterned-ness – in a reliance on what is sometimes referred to as the 'hermeneutic circle' – patterns described derive legitimacy by virtue of the reproducibility of the range of observation(s) made.

EM/CA Research Questions

We must do away with all explanation, and description alone must take its place. (Wittgenstein, 1953, ¶ 109)

The epistemological difficulties of mainstream social science are compounded by the associated conceptual confusion occasioned by starting with imaginary phenomena (such as 'mental illness') and, subsequently, asking 'why?' questions: seeking *explanation*, before having an adequate *description* of the (postulated) phenomena for which an account is sought. That is to say, the social sciences have, by and large, tended to avoid asking 'how (does). . .?' and 'what (is). . .?'

EM/CA is, in contrast, a fundamentally *descriptive* endeavour. To put it very simply, CA studies turn taking because it is there to be studied; EM asks how we successfully wait for buses. EM/CA looks at things like psychotherapy and asks 'how does that work?' This does not mean that EM/CA findings are unavailable for thinking about *why* things are as they are and how things may be different, but that the task is not seeking causal relationships between variables, nor usurping what is properly the province of politics or economics (McHoul, 2008). EM/CA is best suited to asking questions about *how things stand in the world and what are the methodic practices that produce and sustain the social order?* Two brief examples illustrate such questions.

McCabe *et al.* (2002) investigated how psychiatrists interact with 'psychotic' patients. McCabe *et al.* noted that while patients regularly attempted to discuss the content of their 'symptoms', requested explanations and sought help with relationships with others around 'symptoms', doctors were interested in 'symptom' frequency or 'symptoms' under different drug regimes. McCabe *et al.* identified the difficulties caused by these competing agendas: 'when patients did succeed in raising the topic of their concerns, it was often a source of tangible interactional problems . . . [W]hen patients attempted to present their psychotic symptoms as a topic of conversation, the doctors hesitated and avoided answering the patients' questions, indicating reluctance to engage with these concerns' (McCabe *et al.*, 2002, p. 1148). Doctors managed this by laughing. As the authors note: 'In medical interactions, laughter tends to be used more by patients than by doctors, often for delicate interactional tasks. In our study, the doctors' use of laughter seemed to be problematic as a response to serious talk (questions) from the patient and may have indicated embarrassment when faced with such delicate questions from patients' (McCabe *et al.*, 2002, p. 1148).

A further study (McCabe *et al.*, 2004), using the same data set, employed CA to examine the idea that people diagnosed with 'schizophrenia' have an impaired 'theory of mind' (Leitman *et al.*, 2006), that they cannot appreciate the mental states of others and that this produces communication patterns described as 'symptoms'. The study describes how participants displayed that they 'had' a 'theory of mind' in interaction. McCabe *et al*. concluded that, contrary to conventional psychiatric wisdom, 'schizophrenics with ongoing positive and negative symptoms appropriately reported . . . mental states of others and designed their contributions to conversations on the basis of what they thought their communicative partners knew and intended'. In another finding casting doubt on assumptions that 'schizophrenia' entails a failure of 'reality testing', they found that patients' 'psychotic' beliefs were held '*despite the realization* [by patients that] *they are not shared*' (McCabe *et al*., 2004, p. 401).

Such studies, in showing seen-but-unnoticed aspects of interactions between mental health service users and professionals, can tell us a great deal about the priorities and worries of mental health service users; the ways medical consultations (and medical training) might more helpfully be organized to support and respect service users; and the evident – empirically demonstrable – discrepancy between professional beliefs about 'psychosis' and the *actual* capacities of those so diagnosed.

Doing EM/CA: What Kind of Data?

As the key aim is the explication of the 'conversational and other methodic practices whereby members of society assemble social actions' (Maynard & Clayman, 2003, p. 195) EM/CA avoids researcher-generated data. Data obtained by questionnaires, interviews, focus groups and so on are of no use (unless studied as phenomena themselves: 'The Research Interview' becomes topic, not resource).

There are two reasons for this: first, *pace* Schütz (1962), is the epistemological distinction between first and second order *constructs*. Unlike the natural sciences where *first order constructs* account for phenomena such as rocks, trees and capybaras (plate tectonics, photosynthesis and evolution), the social sciences deal not with *objects*, but with *persons* with 'perfectly good and sufficient descriptions of themselves' (McHoul, 2008, p. 4). Replacing such descriptions with *second order constructs* (professional accounts of persons' accounts of themselves) is not only to treat people as cultural dopes, but also to mistake the epistemological status of our object of study – employing procedures developed in the natural sciences to ask questions incommensurable with the methods used (Wittgenstein, 1953).

Secondly, attending to what may be described as 'ecological validity', EM/CA's preference is for naturally occurring, or 'naturally inscribed' materials. Thus, although standard social science suggests that to understand the 'quality of life' of 'intellectually disabled' persons we administer a quality of life questionnaire, to understand how psychotherapy 'works' we interview 'expert' therapists, and to understand public 'beliefs' about mental health we hold a focus group, EM/CA suggests, simply, going directly to the source.

Vast quantities of *professionally unmediated* data on virtually any topic of interest to mental health practitioners are available. Talk about 'quality of life' saturates interactions between people with intellectual disabilities and professionals – even if not described as such (McHoul & Rapley, 2002; Rapley, 2004); the 'nuts and bolts' of psychotherapy are obtainable from therapy transcripts (Peräkylä *et al.*, 2008); public 'beliefs' about mental health can be obtained in any daily newspaper, a copy of *Cosmopolitan*, or by a mouse click on huge numbers of 'self-help' sites on the Internet (Hansen *et al.*, 2003).

Involving Research Participants and Mental Health Service Users

There need be no research participants in the sense that 'participant' is usually understood: EM/CA treats *the already-occurring documentary record of interaction* as data available for analysis. Whether working with naturally inscribed data (case notes, care plans, professional training texts or subsequently transcribed data, such as psychotherapy transcripts), participants need not be directly involved at all. For studies like Goode's (1994) analysis of wards for children with rubella syndrome or Weider's (1974) study of the 'code' in a halfway house, good practice dictates central involvement in project design and management by service users themselves (Stone & Priestley, 1996; see also Chapter 4).

How to use EM/CA

> There are hardly any prescriptions to be followed, if one wants to do 'good CA' (tenHave, 2010).

This example analyses a group cognitive behavioural therapy (CBT) session for people hearing voices.[1] The example shows the detail of Jeffersonian transcription, and how CA is a cumulative enterprise. It is familiarity with the corpus of CA observations of 'social facts' – for example, about conversational structure, prosody and topic management – that enables analysts to comprehend the details of interaction. Speakers are Stuart (S, a 'medication-resistant schizophrenic'), Richard and Mike (R and M, clinical psychologists). Analysis investigated negotiations about therapeutic knowledge, compared to voice hearers' personal accounts.[2] Much of the talk appears less a collaboration than a therapeutic monologue, about how Stuart should understand his 'reality' (see Charles Antaki's website for exercises in transcription and a glossary of transcription symbols at http://www-staff.lboro.ac.uk/~sscal/notation.htm).

Stuart has just been talking about how helpful he finds clozapine in managing his voices. The extract starts with Mike 'asking' to change the subject. With a dysfluent delivery, Mike proposes not an exploration of Stuart's experience, but a therapist-modified reworking of Stuart's prior account.

---

[1] There is an extensive literature on data transcription. For an overview see Jefferson (2004), tenHave (2001, 2007) and exercises at Charles Antaki's website.

[2] A full version is reported in Wise and Rapley (2009).

Extract

```
51  M:  C- (0.2) c'n I j'st (0.5) <zoo:m 'us ↓back to (0.4)
52      that situation la:st ni:[ght ]> (th't-)
53  S:                          [YEH.]
54      (0.6)
55  M:  Um
56      (1.0)
57  M:  ·hh ↑ONE of the things th't impre[ssed m]e:
58  S                                    [  Mm. ]
59      Mmm.=
60  M:  =↓with: um (0.1) the: way: you descri:bed it
61      w'[s]
62  S:    [Y]EH.
63  M:  u↑:m:
64      (1.0)
65  M:  ·hh (0.5) >↑U'm almost thinking it w's- i:t w's
66      kinda like a< ↑three: stage process °with-°
67      (1.0)
68  M:  ↓well (.) more than that I spose [>(hh)< ↑I']
69  S:                                   [Ri:ght↑     ]
70  M:  could ((smiley voice)) >I could build in
71  M:  lo[ts of sta]ges °↓couldn't I-°< ·hh [((cough))]
72  S:    [Right.   ]                        [↑YEAH     ]
73  S:  Yeh.=
74  M:  =↑He[aring- ]
75  M:      [((finger clicking sound))]
76  M:  hear:ing something↑=
77  S:  =Yeh.
78  M:  ((finger clicking sound))= ↓deci:ding whether or
79      not it w's a voi:ce (0.2)
80  S:  Uh huh.
81      (0.5)
82  M:  deci:ding whether it was true or not=
83  S:  =Yeah.
84  M:  and ↑then deciding what
85  M:  [you're gonna do: about i]t
86  S:  [As a voi:ce yeah.       ] >Ye:ah. °As a voice
87  S:      [Mik-°<]
88  M:      [or   ] what your re↑action ↓w's
89  M:  gonn[a be.]
90  S:      [Ye  ]ah (0.1) >that it's gonna be.< (0.1)
91  M:  ↑An[d]
92  S:     [Y]eh.
93  M:  s:- cs:- ↑it kinda sounds quite deliberate ↓the way
94      you descri:be it. (0.5) ↑More than jus' ↓lu:cky
95      <th't i' did-n'> (0.2) sen:d you
```

```
96           cra:z[y  ]
97    S:          [CWA]ZY.  [Yeh.]
98    M:                   [Bu- ]  ↑bu'  (.)  th't you wer[e-]
99    S:                                             [Ye]h.
100          (0.3)
101   M:     ↑It sou:nds like ↓you- (0.2) you were
102          (0.8)
103   M:     ·hhh
104          (1.2)
105   M:     <↑i:n contro:l↑>
106          (0.2)
107   S:     YEAH.
108   M:     ↓and=
109   S:     =Ye:[ah.]
110   M:         [THE] WA:Y YA DESCRIBING IT NO:W is ↓kind of
111          like >priddy< lai:d ↑back ↓about somethi[ng  th]'t
112   S:                                             [Ye:ah.]
113          (0.2)
114   S:     Mmm.
115   M:     ↑could've ↓been quite di↑stre:↓ssing.= ((unctuous
116          sounding))
117   S:     =Mmm.=
118   M:     =W- th- th-=
119   S:     =Mm[m.]
120   M:        [wh]at they were sa:ying:↑
121   S:     Mmm.
122   M:     So: I- I- ↑ya know ↓I just wan'ed t' sa:y
123          (1.3)
124   M:     TALK ABOU:T (0.3) ↑HO:W: (0.4) ↓there seemed to be
125          tho:se <deliberate ↑st [e:ps] ↓'f (0.6) you:
126   S:                           [Mmm.]
127   M:     thinking it throu:gh↑>
128   S:     Mmm.
129          (0.6)
130   M:     which ↑I think we touched on >↓a couple a weeks
131          ago< (.) la: [st week]
132   S:                  [  Mm.  ]
133          (0.2)
134   M:     ·h
135   S:     Mmm.
136          (0.2)
137   M:     b't alSO (0.4) t' sa:y °th't um°=>↑ya know=I'm
138          impressed< by: that (0.3)
139   S:     Yeah.
140          (0.3)
141   M:     <↓because: u:m:> (0.8) [^t] (0.4) ↑SOUNDS LIKE a
142          lot ↓mo:re than luck (0.2) sou[nds li:]ke
```

```
143   S:                                      [Yeh.     ]
144         (0.8)
145   M:   con[↑tro:l]
146   S:      [°Mm.° ]  An'  [↑PI:LLS  (0.1)  as WELL:]
```

Mike's extended turn demonstrates locally operative structures of power asymmetry: it is his 'right' to direct the distribution of talk, topic, and to rewrite Stuart's experience. Stuart, throughout, simply provides agreement tokens – 'mms' and 'yeah's (until, it should be noted, his final turn at line 146). Of particular note, given the diagnosis he has, is Stuart's clear recognition of these conversational realities, and the competent manner in which he displays his awareness of this and also his readiness to accede (e.g., via the overlapping and stressed 'Yeh' precisely timed in anticipation of Mike's utterance in line 53).

Mike's initial hesitancy (lines 54–65) orientates to his revision of Stuart's views. Nevertheless, Mike proposes a 'zoo:m' back to 'that situation la:st ni:ght' (from line 51). The term 'zoo:m', vernacular contractions such as 'c'n' and 'j'st' (line 51), and vague and mitigating terms such as, 'U'm almost thinking' (line 65), 'I spose' (line 68), 'It sou:nds like' (line 101) are instances of the pro-terms (lexical items that stand for other, perhaps more difficult, ones: 'I spose' is, thus, uttered rather than an alternative possibility such as 'I know') which Mike uses to manage the central paradox of CBT: a theoretically 'collaborative' relationship informed by a theory that therapists know better than those whom they are 'treating'.

The pro-terms produce Mike as casual and ordinary, whilst at the same time 'doing therapy' (McHoul & Rapley, 2002). Despite his 'folksy' and *mundane* presentation of phenomena that, by definition, *cannot but be extraordinary*, the essential paradox of CBT leads to the breakdown of Mike's NOT-THERAPIST 'cover identity' (McHoul & Rapley, 2002). Thus, from line 130, Mike refers to material 'which ↑I think we touched on >↓a couple a weeks ago<' in a previous therapy session – but the account Mike gives of 'that situation la:st ni:ght' is, despite the softening devices, structurally akin to *classroom talk* – that is the interaction closely resembles that of TEACHER + PUPIL (McHoul, 1978). Where this leaves *collaboration* in CBT is moot. What is clear, however, is that, Stuart – like the 'patients' in McCabe's studies – displays here an acute social and interactional sensitivity.

Better Quality Studies

Silverman (2010) and many others have written extensively about ensuring the quality of qualitative research (see Chapter 16). Given the family resemblance much EM/CA-inspired work has to discourse analysis (broadly defined) – especially in the areas of MCA and discursive psychology – the injunctions of Antaki *et al.* (2003) are to be commended. In brief, following Atkinson and Heritage (1984), high quality EM/CA work *shows* and *documents* the *intuitively non-apparent competences* that *ordinary speakers use* as they participate in *mutually intelligible, socially organized interaction,* in an *extensive corpus* of *naturally occurring data.*

EM/CA, Mental Health Policy and Future Developments

Although originating in studies of direct relevance to mental health practitioners – Garfinkel's studies of psychiatric interviews (Garfinkel, 1956) and Sacks' work on calls to a suicide helpline – it is only in the last 10–15 years that EM/CA has developed a substantial presence in the analysis of mental health policy and practice.

A body of work has begun to accumulate documenting the methodic practices whereby psychotherapy 'works' – and such analyses of psychotherapeutic practice are well placed to inform current debate about policy initiatives and the relative merits of 'brand name' therapies. EM/CA's contribution is far more than a supplement to traditional 'process' research in psychotherapy: by virtue of its ability to *show psychotherapy happening, as it happens* – rather than, say, providing statistical analyses of therapy ratings – EM/CA can *document* 'brand overlap', the detailed specifics of psychotherapeutic practice-in-interaction and its effects, and can demonstrate – rather than report secondhand – what is experienced as being helpful and effective by service users. Much of this work suggests that the social facticity of notionally distinct therapeutic approaches is less clear-cut than may be suggested by their proponents.

EM/CA has also begun to document the long unappreciated competences of a range of 'client groups'. This work (e.g., McCabe *et al.*, 2002; Rapley & Antaki, 1996, Wise & Rapley, 2009) has suggested that the routine competence of members thought by the mental health professions to be irremediably 'disordered' (people with an intellectual disability or psychosis) is considerably more subtle than contemporary classifications suggest. This work calls into question not only the local, but also the general, meaningfulness of diagnostic categories and offers clear support to the claims of organizations such as the Hearing Voices Network for the democratization of mental health services.

Acknowledgements

I am grateful to Paul tenHave for permission to adapt Box 13.1 from his work. I thank Charles Antaki and Alec McHoul for their continued inspiration, collaboration and friendship. This chapter is for Ella.

References

Antaki, C., Billig, M., Edwards, D. & Potter, J. (2003). Discourse analysis means doing analysis: A critique of six analytic shortcomings. *Discourse Analysis Online*, 1, 1. Retrieved 4 March 2010 from http://extra.shu.ac.uk/daol/articles/v1/n1/a1/antaki2002002.html.

Atkinson, J.M. & Heritage, J. (Eds.) (1984). *Structures of social action: Studies in conversation analysis.* Cambridge: Cambridge University Press.

Carlin, A. (2010). Reading 'A tutorial on membership categorization' by Emanuel Schegloff. *Journal of Pragmatics, 42* (1), 257–261.

Coulter, J. (1979). *The social construction of mind: Studies in ethnomethodology and linguistic philosophy.* London: Macmillan.

Edwards, D. (1995). Sacks and psychology. *Theory and Psychology, 5* (3), 579–597.

Edwards, D. & Potter, J. (1992). *Discursive psychology*. London: Sage.

Garfinkel, H. (1956). Some sociological concepts and methods for psychiatrists. *Psychiatric Research Reports*, 6, 181–198.

Garfinkel, H. (1967). *Studies in ethnomethodology*. Englewood Cliffs, NJ: Prentice-Hall.

Garfinkel, H. (1984). *Studies in ethnomethodology*. Cambridge: Polity.

Garfinkel, H. (2002). *Ethnomethodology's program: Working out Durkheim's aphorism*. Lanham, MD: Rowman & Littlefield.

Garfinkel, H. & Sacks, H. (1970). On formal structures of practical actions. In: J.D. McKinney & E.A. Tiryakian (Eds.) *Theoretical sociology* (pp. 337–66). New York: Appleton Century Crofts.

Goode, D. (1994). *A world without words*. Philadelphia, PA: Temple University Press.

Hansen, S., McHoul, A. & Rapley, M. (2003). *Beyond help: A consumer's guide to psychology*. Ross-on-Wye, PCCS Books.

Heritage, J. (1984). *Garfinkel and ethnomethodology*. Cambridge: Polity Press.

Hester, S. & Eglin, P. (Eds.) (1997). *Culture in action: Studies in membership categorization analysis*. Washington, D.C.: University Press of America.

Jefferson, G. (2004). Glossary of transcript symbols with an introduction. In G. Lerner (Ed). *Conversation analysis: Studies from the first generation* (pp. 13–31). Amsterdam/Philadelphia: John Benjamins.

Leitman, D.I., Ziwich, R., Pasternak, R. & Javitt, D.C. (2006). Theory of mind (ToM) and counterfactuality deficits in schizophrenia: Misperception or misinterpretation? *Psychological Medicine*, 36 (8), 1075–1083.

Leudar, I. & Costall, A. (Eds.) (2009). *Against theory of mind*. Basingstoke: Palgrave Macmillan.

Lynch, M. & Bogen, D. (1996). *The spectacle of history: Speech, text and memory at the Iran-Contra hearings*. Durham, NC: Duke University Press.

Maynard, D.W. & Clayman, S.E. (1991). The diversity of ethnomethodology. In W.R. Scott & J. Blake (Eds.)*Annual Review of Sociology* (vol. 17, pp. 385–418). Palo Alto, CA: Annual Reviews.

Maynard, D.W. & Clayman, S.E. (2003). Ethnomethodology and conversation analysis. In L.T. Reynolds & N.J. Herman-Kinney (Eds.)*The handbook of symbolic interactionism* (pp. 173–202). Walnut Creek, CA: Altamira Press.

McCabe, R., Heath, C., Burns, T. & Priebe, S. (2002). Engagement of patients with psychosis in the consultation: Conversation analytic study. *British Medical Journal*, 325, 1148–1151.

McCabe, R., Leudar, I. & Antaki, C. (2004). Do people with schizophrenia display theory of mind deficits in clinical interactions? *Psychological Medicine*, 34 (3), 401–412.

McHoul, A. (1978). The organization of turns at formal talk in the classroom. *Language in Society*, 7, 183–213.

McHoul, A. (2008). What are we doing when we analyse conversation? Keynote Address, 6th Australasian Symposium on Conversation Analysis and Membership Categorisation Analysis, Brisbane, 5–7 November. Retrieved 14 January 2010 from http://aiemca.net/?page_id=229.

McHoul, A. & Rapley, M. (2000). Sacks and clinical psychology. *Clinical Psychology Forum*, 142, 3–11.

McHoul, A. & Rapley, M. (2002). Should we make a start then?: A strange case of (delayed) client-initiated psychological assessment. *Research on Language and Social Interaction, 35* (1), 73–91.

McHoul, A. & Rapley, M. (2003). What can psychological terms actually do? (Or: if Sigmund calls, tell him it didn't work). *Journal of Pragmatics*, 35 (4), 507–522.

McHoul, A. & Rapley, M. (2005). A case of ADHD diagnosis: Sir Karl and Francis B slug it out on the consulting room floor. *Discourse and Society, 16* (3), 419–449.

Mehan, H. & Wood, H. (1975). *The reality of ethnomethodology.* New York: Wiley.

Moerman, M. (1988). *Talking culture: Ethnography and conversation analysis.* Philadelphia, PA: University of Pennsylvania Press.

Peräkylä, A., Antaki, C., Vehviläinen, S. & Leudar, I. (Eds.) (2008). *Conversation analysis of psychotherapy.* Cambridge: Cambridge University Press.

Potter, J. (2006). Cognition and conversation. *Discourse Studies, 8* (1), 131–140.

Rapley, M. (1998). 'Just an ordinary Australian': Self-categorization and the discursive construction of facticity in 'new racist' political rhetoric. *British Journal of Social Psychology, 37* (3), 325–344.

Rapley, M. (2004). *The social construction of intellectual disability.* Cambridge: Cambridge University Press.

Rapley, M. & Antaki, C. (1996). A conversation analysis of the 'acquiescence' of people with learning disabilities. *Journal of Community and Applied Social Psychology, 6,* 207–227.

Rapley, M., McCarthy, D. & McHoul, A. (2003). Mentality or morality? Membership categories, multiple meanings and mass murder. *British Journal of Social Psychology, 42,* 427–444.

Rapley, M. & McHoul, A. (2002). Self-glorification and its others: The discursive-moral management of sports management. *Journal of Sport and Social Issues, 26* (3), 268–280.

Sacks, H. (1984). Notes on methodology. In J.M. Atkinson & J. Heritage (Eds.) *Structures of social action: Studies in conversation analysis* (pp. 21–27). Cambridge: Cambridge University Press.

Sacks, H. (1992). *Lectures on Conversation* (2 vols). Edited by G. Jefferson with introductions by E.A. Schegloff. Oxford: Basil Blackwell.

Schegloff, E. (2007a). A tutorial on membership categorization. *Journal of Pragmatics, 39* (3), 462–482.

Schegloff, E. (2007b). *Sequence organization in interaction: A primer in conversation analysis* (vol. 1). Cambridge: Cambridge University Press.

Schenkein, J. (1978). Sketch of an analytic mentality for the study of conversational interaction. In J. Schenkein (Ed.) *Studies in the Organization of Conversational Interaction* (pp. 1–6). New York: Academic Press.

Schütz, A. (1962). *Collected papers, Vol. I: The problem of social reality.* The Hague: Martinus Nijhoff.

Sharrock, W. (1995). Ethnographic work. *Discourse Analysis Research Group Newsletter, 11* (1), 3–8.

Silverman, D. (2010) *Doing qualitative research* (3rd edn). London: Sage.

Stone, E. & Priestley, M. (1996). Parasites, pawns and partners: Disability research and the role of non-disabled researchers. *British Journal of Sociology, 47* (4), 699–716.

teMolder, H. & Potter, J. (2005). *Conversation and cognition.* Cambridge: Cambridge University Press.

tenHave, P. (2001). Applied conversation analysis. In A. McHoul & M. Rapley (Eds.) *How to analyse talk in institutional settings: A casebook of methods* (pp. 3–11). London: Continuum.

tenHave, P. (2007). *Doing conversation analysis: A practical guide* (2nd edn). London: Sage.

tenHave, P. (2010). Methodological issues in conversation analysis. Retrieved 14 January 2010 from: http://www2.fmg.uva.nl/emca/mica.htm.

Wieder, D.L. (1974). *Language and social reality: The case of telling the convict code.* The Hague: Mouton.

Wise, M. & Rapley, M. (2009). Cognitive behaviour therapy, psychosis and attributions of irrationality: Or, how to produce cognitions as 'faulty'. *Journal of Critical Psychology, Counselling and Psychotherapy*, Winter, 179–196.

Wittgenstein, L. (1953). *Philosophical investigations* (trans. G.E.M. Anscombe). Oxford: Basil Blackwell.

Wittgenstein, L. (1975). *On certainty*. (G.E.M. Anscombe & G.H. von Wright, Eds; trans. D. Paul & G.E.M. Anscombe). Oxford: Basil Blackwell.

Further reading and useful websites

EM/CA News: Information on Ethnomethodology and Conversation Analysis. http://www2.fmg.uva.nl/emca/sites.htm

Journal of Pragmatics. http://www.elsevier.com/wps/find/journaldescription.cws home/505593/description#description

Research on Language and Social Interaction. http://rolsi.lboro.ac.uk/ROLSIhome.html

14

Q Methodological Research in Mental Health and Psychotherapy

Wendy Stainton Rogers and Phillip O. Dyson

Introduction

In Western society 'hearing voices' is generally taken as a sign of madness. Yet within certain spiritualist groups it is regarded as a 'gift' – the ability to communicate with 'the other side'. Such diametrically opposed understandings of phenomena and issues are part of our everyday experience. Q methodology was created by William Stephenson, specifically as a way to gain insight into the diverse (and often contested) ways in which people – as individuals and as members of groups, communities and other collectivities – make sense of the life-worlds they inhabit. Q methodology offers a very effective means to identify the alternative understandings people have about what 'hearing voices' means, which is why Jones *et al.* (2003) adopted Q methodology to investigate this topic. In this chapter we use their study to 'make real' the ideas and procedures involved in conducting Q methodological research.

Why is it called Q? The answer goes back to a time when statisticians were picking out letters to name their formulations – such as Fisher's *z-scores*. Stephenson arbitrarily chose the letter *q* for his methodology, contrasting it with traditional approaches which he characterized as *r* methodology.

A Short Introduction to Q Methodology

There are two distinctive elements in a Q study: Q-sorting and Q factor analysis (Box 14.1).

Qualitative Research Methods in Mental Health and Psychotherapy: A Guide for Students and Practitioners, First Edition.
Edited by D. Harper and A.R. Thompson.
© 2012 John Wiley & Sons, Ltd. Published 2012 by John Wiley & Sons, Ltd.

Box 14.1 Terminology

Abduction	An alternative logic of inquiry to induction and deduction. The crucial difference is that it is hypothesis *generating* rather than testing
Concourse	All the things that can be said and thought about the topic in question among the population the study is about
Conditions of instruction	Where participants adopt different positions from which to sort – such as 'as I saw things as a teenager', 'how my therapist would see it', 'as I see it when I am happy'
Q-items	Usually statements, selected as a sample of the concourse for the study. These are what are sorted
Q-set	The set of Q items that will be presented to participants
Q-grid	See Figure 14.2
Q-sorting	The process of placing the items of the Q-set into the positions on the Q-grid
Q-sort	The pattern produced when the completed set of items are placed onto the Q-grid and recorded
Q factor analysis	The form of regular factor analysis devised by Stephenson, where it is whole patterns Q-sorting are correlated with each other
Variance	A statistical term indicating how much of the variability in the whole data-set can be 'explained' by the Factor
Exemplificatory Q-sort	Those Q-sorts that only correlate significantly with just one Factor, used (generally with others) as the basis for constructing a 'best estimate' of the sorting pattern for that Factor
Factor account	A short summary outlining the key elements that distinguish the viewpoint or discourse being expressed by the Factor

Q-sorting involves participants ranking items along a dimension like 'most agree' to 'most disagree'. It becomes clearer when you look at what is going on, as shown in Figure 14.1. The participant is placing the items from 'most agree' on his or her right, to 'most disagree' on the left. Participants follow a grid, as shown in Figure 14.2. When completed, the item numbers are recorded in the spaces on the grid. Examples of the sorts of items involved, taken from the 'hearing voices' study, are shown in Table 14.1.

Q factor analysis is a variant on standard factor analysis, With the Q version, the complete sorting pattern of each participant is compared with the sorting patterns of all the other participants. This 'inversion' from the norm allows for a *Gestalt* approach,

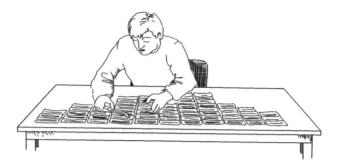

Figure 14.1   Q-sorting.

identifying different points of view about a topic or issue within a particular population. For example, the 'hearing voices' study identified six alternative understandings. One, a *positive spiritual* perspective, differed from the rest because it saw 'hearing voices' as something desirable – a 'gift'. By contrast, the *generic mental illness* perspective drew on the mainstream biomedical understanding of 'madness'.

To understand Q you need to understand the difference between traditional and Q factor analysis. Traditional factor analysis was developed for studies investigating 'traits' – such as whether intelligence is a single capacity of 'cleverness' or is made up of separate traits like 'cleverness with words' and 'mathematical ability' each independent of the other. If just one factor is identified, this indicates that intelligence is a single capacity. But if several different factors are found, this indicates that, say, verbal intelligence and mathematical intelligence are two separate capabilities. In this approach, large numbers of people are given tests to perform, each one designed to tap a different kind of ability. The data, when entered into the factor analysis programme, would look like Table 14.2, although in real life there would be much more of it.

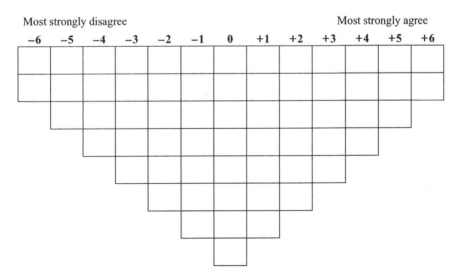

Figure 14.2   The Q response grid.

Table 14.1   Example items from Jones *et al.*'s (2003) hearing voices study.

Item number	Statement
2	People who hear voices are making contact with a different spiritual plane of reality
25	Hearing voices results from being mentally injured as a child
12	Untreated voice hearers are a risk to society
16	Voices can help a person take action that they have lacked the courage to perform

Factor analysis here begins with correlating the scores on the different tests and looking for clusters of tests that are highly correlated. Working systematically to parcel up the inter-correlating tests into clusters, factor analysis first identifies and extracts from the calculation the cluster that explains most of the variance in the data set – Factor 1. The analysis then moves on to account for the variance that is left, again seeking the cluster of inter-correlation that explains the most variance within this depleted set – Factor 2. Although this process continues until all the variance is accounted for, researchers usually stop looking for factors once they become no longer informative.

Q factor analysis works in the same sort of way, but there is a crucial difference. The numbers indicating the placement of items in the Q-sort are not keyed in as though they are the results of 'tests'. Instead, the placement is reversed, as shown in Table 14.3, although again, there would be much more data. Thus, Q factor analysis is not 'by person' but rather 'by sorting pattern'. People are not the 'exemplars', their Q-sorts are.

Q is often regarded as a quantitative method (McKeown & Thomas, 1988), mostly because it uses numbers. But the numbers are not used to *measure* anything; they are ordinal, arising from rank ordering items. Q shares a common purpose with more easily recognizable qualitative approaches like those taken by narrative, discourse an-alytic and phenomenological research. Its goals and underpinning ontological and epistemological assumptions are qualitative in nature.

History

Stephenson invented Q methodology and established it in a letter to *Nature* in 1935. In it he claimed that by inverting the usual way factor analysis is carried out, various novel and valuable insights become possible. Stephenson was not the first to try this

Table 14.2   In a traditional factor analysis, the items are the variables.

People	Test scores			
	Verbal test 1	Verbal test 2	Maths test 1	Maths test 2
Jane	15	19	8	11
Maya	3	8	9	5
Olu	20	19	10	18

Table 14.3   In a Q factor analysis, the participants are the variables.

Q-sort items	Q-sort placement of item		
	Beth's Q-sort	Dan's Q-sort	Delia's Q-sort
1. Given the right circumstances, most of us would hear voices	+1	−4	−1
2. People who hear voices are making contact with a different spiritual plane of reality	+4	−3	0
3. People hear voices when the Devil or other evil spirit possesses them	−2	0	−5
4. Hearing voices is a life-long condition	0	+2	−2

version of factor analysis, but he was the first to recognize its real potential. Kohlberg (Stephenson's student and then research assistant at the University of Chicago) describes how: '[b]ehind the details of Q technique, many of us got the sense of a general logic of discovery, hypothesis formation and classification that needed exploration. ... Q technique opened up ... the logic of the humanities, the logic of interpretation of art and literature' (Zangwill *et al.*, 1972, p. xiii).

Stephenson, pretty well throughout his life, was seen as an irascible rebel and was seldom understood. When he moved on from Chicago to Missouri (by way of a short spell in the advertising industry), his interests turned to the study of communication, public opinion and advertising. Here he took the maverick stance of viewing the mass media not as agents of entertainment but of persuasion, and, thereby, as forms of social control: 'In our theoretical framework one doesn't seek to educate people, or inform them about matters; instead one sets about getting them to change their *behaviour* in such a way that there will be a concurrent change in attitude; the latter will be consequential' (Stephenson, 1967, p. 2).

Both theoretically and methodologically, his were not popular positions to adopt in an academic establishment dominated by hypothetico-deductive thinking and quantitative methods. It is hardly surprising that in his lifetime Stephenson's authority gradually faded. He went from being a key player in the establishment of psychology as a discipline, director of the newly formed Institute of Experimental Psychology at the University of Oxford in the 1940s, to a lowly (but much revered) professor of journalism in a relatively obscure university in the United States. But with the emergence of critical psychology, he is once again gaining real respect among psychologists.

(Post)Modern times

These days Q research is flourishing, albeit increasingly outside the United States where the stranglehold of quantitative approaches is still strong. Stephenson died in 1989 but his influence endures, especially through the work of his graduate students. Most important of these scholars has undoubtedly been Steven R. Brown, whose book,

Political Subjectivity (Brown, 1980), is the standard text for anyone starting out in Q research. As we write it is Brown who maintains and sustains the Q-METHOD discussion list (q-method@listserv.kent.edu), constantly updates the Q research bibliography, and has taken Q around the world, with groups of Q methodologists highly active in Norway, South America and South Korea to name but some. He instigated the *International Society for the Scientific Study of Subjectivity* (ISSSS), which has an annual conference and a journal, *Operant Subjectivity*.

In the year of his death, Stephenson gave the keynote lecture at an Economic and Social Research Council (ESRC) funded seminar on Q methodology at Reading University in England, organized by a group of people writing as a communal author called Beryl Curt, who had discovered, in Q, a method for studying 'textuality and tectonics': 'What we were looking for, as a method, was the "opposite" of correlating "traits", something which correlated whole structures of readings (e.g. about people) in order to disclose how they "shake out" into sets of very similar accounts, i.e. shared stories' (Curt, 1994, pp. 119–120).

The outcome has been the development of Q as a 'discursive, constructivist, and hence as an essentially qualitative method' (Stenner *et al.*, 2009). Q, in this context, becomes a form of discourse analysis (Curt, 1994, p. 128; R. Stainton Rogers, 1995; W. Stainton Rogers, 1991, 1997/1998). There are certainly differences between the approaches to, and readings of, what Q methodology 'is' and 'is for' (see e.g., Stainton Rogers & Stainton Rogers, 1990). But there remains a common purpose, which is to conduct and promote Q methodology as a potent and unique way of carrying out research, with enormous potential to impact upon theory, policy and practice as well as making substantial contributions to our knowledge and understanding.

Epistemological Assumptions

Stephenson rejected the epistemological assumptions of traditional factor analysis – that 'everyone has every psychological attribute to some degree'. This, he argued, 'is both unnecessary for scientific purposes and incapable of any proof' (Stephenson, 1953, p. 3). Stephenson actually based his 'challenge' to the Newtonian tradition in psychology on epistemological and ontological presumptions (as well as mathematics) that were more familiarly associated with the quantum mechanics of physics (see Watts & Stenner, 2003).

However, early in its history, Q-sorting became appropriated by those who sought to 'improve' the technique so that it could be used to measure such things as the impact of therapy and to 'assess personality'. Block devised a standardized Q-set (the 'California Q-set'; Block, 1961, 2008) which he used to compare individuals' sorting patterns to templates (such as 'well adjusted' compared with 'maladjusted') and in this way to determine their state of mental health. In many parts of the psychotherapy research community it is Block's version that is popularly known and used.

Whatever the merits (or not) of using Q-sorting in this way, it is based on epistemological and ontological assumptions that are contrary to what Stephenson intended for

Q. Block's use of Q was based on his belief that 'normality' was something that could be objectively measured. Stephenson made it absolutely clear that Q was not intended to measure anything.

Q methodology is best known as a way of studying *subjectivity*, at least within the overall Q community. Q enables people to express their own perceptions of their personal subjectivity, such as what it feels like to experience depression. It allows such subjective aspects to be mapped out in fine detail, providing researchers with a novel and powerful tool for interrogating subjective experience. Q is often used like this by psychotherapists to conduct fine-grained, case study investigations of an individual's subjective experiences, self-perceptions, aspirations and the like, mapping out their client's subjectivity over time and across various aspects of their emotional and cognitive mental life. Here the Q-set is drawn from statements made in therapy sessions. Goldstein and Goldstein (2005) did so to investigate the subjective self-esteem of a client they call L. Having constructed a self-esteem Q-set from her own conversations and writings, they had her carry out 12 Q-sorts under different conditions of instruction, including 'the way I am as a parent' and 'when I was divorced'. Four quite different self-perceptions were found. These were then fed back to L in subsequent therapy sessions, enabling her to become more self-aware and, hence, more able to resolve some of the issues for which she had sought therapy.

However, once Q is couched within a social constructionist epistemology, it provides a powerful technique for studying *inter-subjectivity*: how argument and truth-claims are deployed within and between the competing positions taken by groups with different stakes to claim, statuses to defend, values to endorse and realities to construct. It enables us to conduct an analysis of discourse where knowledge is not seen as in any way absolute, but multiple and contingent on time and place and purpose. Crucially, Q specifically expects people to express different opinions in their Q-sorting – as did L in the Goldstein and Goldstein study under different conditions of instruction. Q-sorts are simply a way to express one or more discursive position(s). It is the textuality and tectonics operating through and between discourses that are under scrutiny in a Q study.

Research Questions

Among researchers who, like ourselves, adopt a social constructionist stance, Q studies are primarily used to find out about 'what is going on' in the conversations and other forms of social interplay operating *between* people – including communicative processes such as education, journalism, advertising, entertainment and, these days, increasingly through people's interactions on the Internet and in the virtual worlds made possible by it. Here, Q methodology is being used less as a means to interrogate individual subjectivities and more as a taxonomic tool. It is more like the field trip where an ecologist ventures into unknown territory to identify and describe the various plants and animals that occupy it. Q can similarly be used to map out the terrain of possible/culturally available viewpoints on a topic. Done this way, a Q study explores the complex interplays among and between the discourses occupying the various niches within a discursive eco-system, discovering how the operations of each one determines the ecological niches available for others to occupy. Or, taking a geological analogy, alternative discourses can be seen as operating like tectonic plates, in constant flux, moulding and shaping one another. Q can enable us to name and depict the textuality of the discourses in play and, through further interpretation, to map out their tectonic relations to each other (Curt, 1994).

Within such an epistemology, research questions are minimalist and open-ended, posing questions like: What is going on here? What different versions of reality are in play? Which ones are dominant, which ones hidden? How is power being exercised? By whom, and for what purposes?

Such questions are abductive (i.e., hypothesis generating rather than testing). Abductive research is about concentrating on what is puzzling, unexpected or contradictory in the data, rather than looking for systematic lawfulness. Abductive methods expose riddles and mysteries, the solving of which offer insights that can be used to 'make sense' of 'what is going on'. Q is particularly useful for abductive research. While some factors are easy to understand, most Q studies generate at least one factor that is a real conundrum. The sorting pattern presents a mix of ideas that are unfamiliar to the researchers, making it hard to find any coherence in what is being expressed. Deciphering factors like this is a matter of actively striving for meaning – for example, by interviewing the people whose Q-sorts were exemplificatory. It is this that makes Q methodology such an effective abductive method (for others see Shank, 1998). Almost always a Q study depicts one or more discourse that the researcher(s) *did not* know about or understand, or, at least, one that hovers on the boundary of understanding. This is much less a feature of other qualitative methods, where only those themes, for example, that the researcher recognizes are included in the interpretation.

What Kind of Data are Most Appropriate for Q Methodological Studies?

Posters, paintings and photographs have all been used as items, but statements are by far the most usual. Selecting statements for a Q-set is a lengthy and careful procedure because this is where sampling is done. The Q-set provides as good a sample as possible of what Q methodologists call the 'concourse': all the things that can be said and thought about the topic in question among the participant population selected for study. Researchers must make sure all participants in the study are able, in sorting the Q-set, to give a reasonable account of their own viewpoint. However, the Q-set must also be kept to a manageable size, usually somewhere between 30 and 80 statements, although among Q researchers opinions differ about the optimum balance between a 'good' sample of the concourse and a 'manageable' number of items to sort. Each item is randomly numbered for recording purposes.

Increasingly, Q studies are conducted as part of a mixed methods inquiry, and designing the Q-set is informed by procedures such as interviewing, focus groups, ethnography (in 'real life' and on the Internet) and media analysis (including relevant texts of all kinds including films and novels as well as the academic literature in the field). Sampling is often at least partially theoretically informed. Jones *et al.* (2003) made sure they included a range of items within three broad categories of items: biomedical explanations, psychological and spiritual.

Participants in a Q study are not to be chosen as 'representative' (as noted earlier, sampling is done on the concourse) but *strategically* – to optimize opportunities for disparate discourses to be identified. The selection is informed by the research question and the population under scrutiny. Jones *et al.* (2003) chose to concentrate on voice hearers, and looked for a broad representation of those receiving and those not receiving mental health treatment and including members of charismatic Christian and Spiritualist communities.

Involving Research Participants and Service Users

Participants (whether they be mental health service users or not) can be involved at each stage of the Q process. P.O.D.'s research on self-harm is a good example of how innovative recruitment strategies can engage with participants differently. Using social networking sites in ways that are ethical has enabled him to recruit much more widely and target recruitment more effectively. Recruiting via email lists identified several people with experience of self-harm who were enthusiastic about feeding into and participating in the research. Gaining access to a greater variety of participants really maximizes the taxonomic potential of Q and the benefits of increased anonymity in this setting can encourage 'harder to reach' participants to take part in the research.

One of the ways in which Q methodology studies differ from other qualitative research is that, as a range of stories are to be investigated, participants are often recruited from a range of stakeholder groups – for example, both service users and professionals (Dudley *et al.*, 2009; James & Warner, 2005; Warner, 2008). The accounts of these different groups are accorded equal epistemological value. Sometimes, interviews with participants provide the material from which the Q items are drawn and they may provide initial feedback on the Q-set, refining the number and phrasing of statements. Participants may also be involved in the piloting and subsequent completion of the Q-sorts, ensuring that their perspectives are included in the data generation. Inclusion does not end there; participants can support data-analysis/interpretation. In a number of Q methodology studies, participants are interviewed about their sorting pattern. As with other approaches, service users may also be involved as part of the project management group or as members of an external reference group.

How to Perform a Q Methodological Study

Q methodology is carried out in discrete stages. Stenner *et al.* (2009) provide more detail than space here allows.

Q-set

Selecting the right language for the statements needs to be done carefully and systematically, following the principles of good questionnaire design. For example, each statement should express a single idea, negatives must be avoided (as they pose problems if sorted in negative categories) and the language must be accessible and appropriate for the participants. With suitably simple language and relatively low numbers of statements, Q studies have been carried out that include as participants quite young children and people with learning disabilities (McKenzie, 2009).

It is usual to get feedback on an initial sample of items, usually two or three times as many as needed for the Q-set. Feedback is sought on whether there is a numerical balance between statements likely to be agreed or disagreed with, whether they are easy to understand and whether any items are duplicated or omitted. This feedback helps us to refine the items, reduce them and work towards a rough balance of positive and negative statements. It is good practice, where possible, to pilot test the Q-set, running a full analysis to identify items that are good and poor discriminators. This allows for a final fine-tuning of the Q-set.

Q-grid

The grid pattern is a means to standardize responses, which makes the analysis more straightforward, but, most importantly, it makes the task of ranking large numbers of items manageable. It is relatively easy to simply rank order up to about 20 statements in a long line. More than that becomes difficult. Using a grid as shown in Figure 14.2 makes the task relatively easy to do. The grid design is dependent on the number of items in the Q-sort, and the degree of differentiation required, although researchers seldom use more than 13 categories (−6 to +6).

Collecting the data

The study begins with the strategic selection and recruitment of participants.

Q-sorting   Traditionally, sorters were provided with each item on a small card or slip of paper of a manageable size (see Figure 14.1) and many Q researchers still do this. However, there is now a choice of software that delivers the sorting task online, usually in a series of binary choices. The end result is the same – a numeric record of the items that have been placed in a pre-specified grid pattern as shown in Figure 14.3. Each statement is given a number and it is this number that is entered into the grid.

There are no set rules about how to deliver and receive back Q-sorts (personally, by post, online, etc.). Participants can sort on their own or as a group and with or without the researcher present. Each method has advantages and disadvantages. Response rates differ in similar ways to standard questionnaire research, often with lower returns as Q-sorting is demanding and time-consuming. Usually, a few sorts are returned incorrectly coded or with data missing. These are usually excluded from the data.

Most strongly disagree   Most strongly agree

−6	−5	−4	−3	−2	−1	0	+1	+2	+3	+4	+5	+6
1	6	26	30	5	2	18	3	19	23	16	4	12
32	7	31	38	8	10	22	20	46	36	24	13	52
	9	37	44	15	11	28	25	48	39	27	47	
		51	45	41	14	34	29	50	42	33		
			55	49	17	35	43	56	53			
				58	21	40	60	59				
					62	54	61					
						57						

Figure 14.3 A Q grid completed.

Additional information Many Q researchers seek additional information from participants to help in factor interpretation. It is usual (but not essential) to gather demographic information (e.g., gender, age) although other information may be more relevant (such as membership of a church or use of mental health services) and should be gathered. Some researchers observe participants sorting and interview them afterwards. Others gather written comments on reasons for item placement, interpretation, and so on. One approach that works well is to directly ask participants what they think has influenced their views.

Statistical analysis

The next step is for data from the completed grids to be entered into appropriate software for analysis. This can be done using a package such as SPSS for the factor analysis with some additional calculation. Q researchers these days mostly use dedicated software programs such as *PQmethod* (http://www.lrz.de/~schmolck/qmethod/index.htm) and *PCQ for Windows* (www.pcqsoft.com/) to perform the statistical analysis. These offer a range of choices about the ways in which the data can be manipulated and described. Other software delivers Q-sorts online and then performs the analysis (see below).

All three strategies yield the same basic output – a number of factors are identified, together with a 'best estimate' of the Q-sort associated with that factor. Each depicts a holistic pattern of response, from which the particular viewpoint or discourse can be interpreted.

These are arrived at in three stages. First, the *factors are established* through a sequence of calculations involving correlation and data rotation. Different statistical procedures are possible, each with its own advocates in the Q community. Many Q researchers simply use the software following a standardized procedure which makes all the choices for them. Others prefer to 'play around' with the data in different ways in order to achieve particular outcomes. Next, *exemplificatory Q-sorts are selected* for each of the factors – these are the ones that correlate significantly with just *this* factor. Here 'significance level' is selected much as in more familiar tests of statistical significance. Finally, a weighting procedure is used to *generate a 'best estimate' Q-sort* for that factor. It is usual at this stage to do some preparatory interpretation, to identify the factors to be interpreted.

Brown (1980) and Watts and Stenner (2005) are both good places to start in understanding the technicalities of this statistical analysis. However, if statistics are not your forte, do not worry. The software packages will do these stages for you, offering you more or less choice about what strategies to use. There is also advice and help available on the QMETHOD list, and a growing number of off- and online tutorials and workshops.

Interpreting the factors

In Q, interpretation is similar to the way researchers 'immerse themselves' in the data in other thematic, discourse or narrative analytic interpretations. The Q-sort for each factor is the starting point for the next stage – producing a factor account (sometimes called explication or exegesis), one for each of the factors chosen for further interpretation. Not all factors need to be interpreted (although there are disputes among Q researchers about when to stop). When writing for a doctorate or publication where space is at a premium, it is good to be selective, and aim to tell a good story around just some factors, preferably those most relevant to the research question. Each factor account summarizes the key elements of the viewpoint expressed.

Next comes an exploration of the significance of the viewpoint, its origins and the influences that have shaped it, as well as its implications and/or applications. Interpretation involves drawing on a whole range of information: common characteristics among the people whose Q-sorts were exemplificatory, explanations for why certain items are placed in one column rather than another, accounts from the literature, expressing the same argument. Shank (1998) identifies this as researchers making use of the sense-making skills that all of us develop through our life experiences, and use every day to navigate through and manage our relationships and our lives.

In Q research it is usual to give each factor a label, and they can be re-ordered if this makes for a more coherent account. This is possible because the order of the factors can be arbitrary. The amount of variance explained may well be as much of a reflection of the participants selected as the relative popularity or importance of the viewpoint expressed. For instance, in W.S.R.'s study of explanations for health and illness (Stainton Rogers, 1991) Factor 1 was all about the role of 'willpower' – spiritual strength to maintain health and fend off disease, a relatively rare understanding. Its ranking was an artefact, arising from the disproportionate number of 'alternative' practitioners among the participants in the study.

Principles of a Good Q Study

Good Q studies identify a number of clearly alternative viewpoints on the matter in question. The Q-set is well designed: comprehensive of 'what is said and thought', each item expressing a single opinion or depiction, in language accessible to and appropriate for the diversity of participants included. Preparation is thorough and thoughtful, to ensure this quality. Interpretation is equally insightful and done with a determination to recognize and solve the riddles presented by hard-to-interpret factors. Often the best studies are done collectively, bringing a diversity of experience and expertise, especially to the tasks of designing the Q-set and interpreting the factors.

Technically speaking, there is a fair amount of debate between Q researchers about the 'best' way to do it. Possibly what matters more is to give a clear account of what you have done, the choices you have made, and back these up with an informed justification of 'doing it your way'. It is important to follow appropriate research principles such as those used in questionnaire design and thematic analysis. What every Q researcher agrees you *cannot* do is to make claims that are unjustified by the method (such as it being able to tap into every alternative viewpoint) or the analysis (claiming you can say anything about what proportion of the population hold particular views).

Q Methodology and Policy

We have noted in the chapter how Q methodological studies can be used in a range of ways which may impact on mental health theory, policy and practice. This can occur at both the micro and macro levels of policy. For example, at the micro level, when completing a Q-sort participants must resolve a whole range of differing (sometimes conflicting) ideas, emotions and concerns. A number of researchers have capitalized upon this to use Q-sorting as an aid to reflexive practice. McKeown *et al.* (1999) used just such an approach to investigate the alternative ways that mental health professionals thought risk should be managed in mental health services. Their Q methodological study was not only a piece of research, but they also utilized the Q-sort as part of a training programme for managers working in the service. Completing the Q-sort allowed these managers to grapple with the contradictions and ambiguities they faced when considering how the service should be run.

Because Q excels at identifying the range of ways in which an issue can be conceived, it can help, at the macro level, to question some of the taken-for-granted assumptions underlying social policy. For example, a historical perspective on how current notions of childhood are constructed (Stainton Rogers & Stainton Rogers, 1992) can lead into alternative perspectives on child protection policies (Stainton Rogers *et al.*, 1992). Similarly, examining the range of ways in which women's mental health is storied in relation to sexual abuse can also help us to rethink the provision of mental health services (Warner, 2008).

Recent Innovation in Q Research

Historically, Q-sorts have had the same difficulties in administration as had questionnaires prior to the advent of websites such as surveymonkey.com. Q-sorting began as a manual paper-based task. Then email became useful for sending and receiving Q-sets and grids. Now online 'Flash' and 'Java script' programs (developed for games and chatrooms) are changing this. Websites such as WebQ (http://www.lrzmuenchen.de/~schmolck/qmethod/webq/) and FlashQ (http://www.hackert.biz/flashq/home/) now provide Q researchers with an opportunity to administer Q-sorts online. Both are available as free downloads.

Internet and other new technological developments in communication are making it easier for Q researchers to work across national and language boundaries, for instance in translating Q-sets for each other in order to extend the linguistic and cultural diversity of the participants in a study. There may be problems with cross-cultural work, given that participant recruitment strategies may have more influence than 'culture' in different sites. But these simply mean one should take extra care when making claims about the study. Similarly, the massively improved access to images and music available to us are likely to open up the kinds of item-sets we can use.

New technologies will undoubtedly enhance the user experience of Q methodology – such as touch-screen technology, improved graphics and 3-D (which could be great fun for doing 'hand rotation' of factors). Where this will lead we cannot tell, but as Q methodology increases in popularity, new participant-friendly approaches for Q-sorting will undoubtedly emerge. The technological future for Q is bright. As Star Trek's Spock would say, what we have to do now is 'go forth and prosper'.

References

Block, (1961). *The Q-sort method in personality assessment and psychiatric research*. Springfield, IL: Charles Thomas.

Block, J. (2008). *The Q-sort in character appraisal: Encoding subjective impressions of persons quantitatively*. Washington, D.C.: APA Books.

Brown, S. (1980). *Political subjectivity: Applications of Q methodology in political science*. New Haven, CT: Yale University Press.

Curt, B. (1994). *Textuality and tectonics: Troubling social and psychological research*. Buckingham: Open University Press.

Dudley, R., Siitarinen, J., James, I. & Dodgson, G. (2009). What do people with psychosis think caused their psychosis? A Q methodology study. *Behavioural and Cognitive Psychotherapy*, 37, 11–24.

Goldstein, D.M. & Goldstein, S.E. (2005). Q methodology study of a person in individual therapy. *Clinical Case Studies*, 4 (1), 40–56.

James, M. & Warner, S. (2005). Coping with their lives: Women, learning disabilities, self-harm and the secure unit – A Q-methodological study. *British Journal of Learning Disabilities*, 33, 120–127.

Jones, S., Guy, A. & Omrod, J.A. (2003). A Q-methodological study of hearing voices: A preliminary exploration of voice hearers' understanding of their experiences. *Psychology and Psychotherapy: Theory, Research and Practice, 76*, 189–209.

McKenzie, J.A. (2009). Constructing the intellectually disabled person as a subject of education: A discourse analysis using Q methodology. Doctoral dissertation, University of Grahamstown, South Africa.

McKeown, B. & Thomas, D. (1988). *Q methodology.* Beverley Hills, CA: Sage.

McKeown, M., Hinks, M., Stowell-Smith, M., Mercer, D. & Forster, J. (1999). Q methodology, risk training and quality management. *International Journal of Health Care Quality Assurance, 6* (12), 254–266.

Shank, G. (1998). The extraordinary powers of abductive reasoning. *Theory and Psychology, 8* (6), 841–860.

Stainton Rogers, R. (1995). Q methodology. In J.A. Smith, R. Harré & L. Van Langenhove (Eds.)*Rethinking methods in psychology* (pp. 178–192). London: Sage.

Stainton Rogers, R. & Stainton Rogers, W. (1990). What the Brits got out of the Q and why their way may not line up with the American way of getting into it! *EJC/REC 1* (1) 1990. Retrieved 22 August 2010 from: http://www.cios.org/EJCPUBLIC/001/1/00113.html.

Stainton Rogers, R. & Stainton Rogers, W. (1992). *Stories of childhood: Shifting agendas in child concern.* London: Prentice Hall.

Stainton Rogers, W. (1991). *Explaining health and illness: An exploration of diversity.* Hemel Hempstead: Harvester Wheatsheaf.

Stainton Rogers, W. (1997/1998). Using Q as a form of discourse analysis, special edition. *Operant Subjectivity, 21* (1/2).

Stainton Rogers, W., Hevey, D. & Ash, E. (Eds.) (1992). *Child abuse and neglect: Facing the challenge* (2nd edn). London: Batsford.

Stenner, P., Watts, S. & Worrell, M. (2009). Q methodology. In C. Willig & W. Stainton Rogers (Eds.)*The Sage handbook of qualitative methods in psychology* (pp. 215–239). London: Sage.

Stephenson, W. (1953). *The study of behavior.* Chicago: University of Chicago Press.

Stephenson, W. (1967). *The play theory of mass communication.* Chicago: University of Chicago Press.

Warner, S. (2008). *Understanding the effects of child sexual abuse: Feminist revolutions in theory, research and practice.* London: Routledge.

Watts, S. & Stenner, P. (2003). Q methodology, quantum theory and psychology. *Operant Subjectivity, 26*, 155–173.

Watts, S. & Stenner, P. (2005). Doing Q methodology: Theory, method and interpretation. *Qualitative Research in Psychology, 2*, 67–91.

Zangwill, O.L., Kohlberg, L. & Brenner, D.J. (1972). Introduction, William Stephenson. In S.R. Brown & D.J. Brenner (Eds.)*Science, psychology, and communication: Essays honoring William Stephenson* (pp. ix–xxv). New York: Teachers College Press.

Further reading

Jones, S., Guy, A. & Omrod, J.A. (2003). A Q-methodological study of hearing voices: A preliminary exploration of voice hearers' understanding of their experiences. *Psychology and Psychotherapy: Theory, Research and Practice, 76*, 189–209.

Stenner, P., Watts, S. & Worrell, M. (2009). Q methodology. In C. Willig & W. Stainton Rogers (Eds.) *The Sage handbook of qualitative methods in psychology* (pp. 215–239). London: Sage.

Watts, S. & Stenner, P. (2005). Doing Q methodology: Theory, method and interpretation. *Qualitative Research in Psychology, 2*, 67–91.

15

Thematic Analysis

Helene Joffe

Description of the Method

Thematic analysis (TA) is a method for identifying and analysing patterns of meaning in a data set (Braun & Clarke, 2006). It illustrates which themes are important in the description of the phenomenon under study (Daly *et al.*, 1997). The end result of a TA should highlight the most salient constellations of meanings present in the data set. Such constellations include affective, cognitive and symbolic dimensions. If one were looking at how those who do not take up the services of mental health professionals view them, for example, a TA of interviews with a carefully chosen sample of such people would reveal how they represent the various mental health professionals. This, in turn, would reveal what keeps them away from the services offered by those such as psychotherapists and psychologists. Thus, a TA can tap the manifest and latent drivers concerning an issue such as uptake of mental health professional services.

Because a TA refers to themes, the notion of a theme must be examined more closely. A theme refers to a specific pattern of meaning found in the data. It can contain *manifest* content – that is, something directly observable such as mentions of stigma across a series of interview transcripts. Alternatively, it can contain more *latent* content, such as references in the transcripts, which refer to stigma implicitly, via mentions of maintaining social distance from a particular group, such as certain mental health professionals. Specific criteria need to be stipulated concerning what can and cannot be coded within such themes; otherwise this form of content is highly subjective. Themes are thus patterns of explicit and implicit content. TAs tend to draw on both types of theme. Often one can identify a set of manifest themes, which point to a more latent

Qualitative Research Methods in Mental Health and Psychotherapy: A Guide for Students and Practitioners, First Edition.
Edited by D. Harper and A.R. Thompson.
© 2012 John Wiley & Sons, Ltd. Published 2012 by John Wiley & Sons, Ltd.

level of meaning. The deduction of latent meanings underpinning sets of manifest themes requires interpretation (Joffe & Yardley, 2004).

A further important distinction in terms of the demarcation of a theme is whether it is drawn from a *theoretical* idea that the researcher brings to the research (termed deductive) or from the *raw data* itself (termed inductive). While theoretically derived themes allow researchers to replicate, extend and refute existing studies (Boyatzis, 1998), there is little point in conducting qualitative work if one does not want to draw on the naturalistically occurring themes evident in the data. So one utilizes the two together – one goes to the data with certain preconceived categories derived from theories, yet one also remains open to new concepts that emerge. It is important to approach each data set with knowledge of previous findings in the area under study to avoid 're-inventing the wheel'. However, in addition, one wants to take seriously findings that do not match with previous frames and have the potential to revolutionize knowledge of the topic under investigation. Thus, a dual deductive–inductive and latent–manifest set of themes are used together in high-quality qualitative work.

TA has recently been recognized as a method in its own right. Previously, it was widely used in psychology and beyond, often without acknowledgement or demarcation (Boyatzis, 1998; Braun & Clarke, 2006). It has also been used in this way in the evaluation of mental health services. Some argue that the ability to thematize meaning is a necessary generic skill that generalizes across qualitative work (Holloway & Todres, 2003). Like other qualitative methods, TA facilitates the gleaning of knowledge of the meaning made of the phenomenon under study by the groups studied and provides the necessary groundwork for establishing valid models of human thinking, feeling and behaviour. However, TA is among the most systematic and transparent forms of such work, partly because it holds the prevalence of themes to be so important, without sacrificing depth of analysis. Thus, TA not only forms the implicit basis of much other qualitative work, it strives to provide the more systematic transparent form of it.

Historical Origins and Influences

TA is rooted in the much older tradition of content analysis (CA). TA shares many of the principles and procedures of CA, a historically quantitative tradition that dates back to the early twentieth century within the social sciences, but further back in the humanities (Smith, 2000). CA involves establishing categories and then counting the number of instances in which they are used in a text or image. It determines the frequency of the occurrence of particular categories. Many CAs rely purely on counting attributes in data (e.g., particular words or images). CA is appealing because it offers a model for systematic analysis of both elicited and naturally occurring data. It has been widely used for the analysis of mass media material. However, the results it generates have been judged as 'trite' (Silverman, 1993) when they rely exclusively on the frequency outcomes it generates. It is also accused of removing codes from their context, thereby stripping data of its meaning.

The concept of 'thematic analysis' was developed, in part, to go beyond observable material to more implicit, tacit themes and thematic structures (Merton, 1975). For the founder of TA, Gerald Horton, such material can be termed 'themata' and these tacit preferences or commitments to certain kinds of concepts are shared in groups, without conscious recognition of them.

Ideally, contemporary TA is able to offer the systematic element characteristic of CA, but also permits the researcher to combine analysis of the frequency of codes with analysis of their more tacit meanings, thus adding the advantages of the subtlety and complexity of phenomenological pursuits.

Key Epistemological Assumptions

TA is not tied to a particular theoretical outlook and so can be applied when using a range of theories and epistemological approaches. It is well suited to use with social phenomenology (see Fereday & Muir-Cochrane, 2006) as well as with social represen-tations theory (SRT; see Farr & Moscovici, 1984; Joffe, Washer & Solberg, in press). It is well matched to theories with weak constructionist tenets like SRT (Lupton, 1999). Weak constructionism assumes that how people engage with a particular issue is so-cially constructed although the issues themselves have a material basis. This is broadly in keeping with the critical realist position, although with a less dichotomous view concerning the need to be *either* realist *or* social constructionist. In addition, many of the tenets of phenomenology are compatible with weak constructionism (see Willig, in press). A key feature of SRT is that it focuses on the content of people's thoughts/feelings regarding the issue under study without reference to the 'reality' of the issue. For ex-ample, regarding lay conceptualizations of a health service professional, the concern is not with the accuracy of the representation but with what meanings people attach to this profession and the consequences of such meanings for themselves, for others and for the society.

TA serves as a useful tool to illuminate the process of social construction. In particular, combining TAs of a range of data can trace how a particular representation develops. Mass media material (both text and image) can be thematically analysed in parallel to the TA of interviews with lay people and professional groups to examine the circulation and transformation of representations in the process of communication. Unlike cognitive approaches, which do not generally take into account the symbolic meanings that people attach to issues (Lupton, 1999), SRT in combination with TA can provide an inroad into these symbolic meanings.

Symbolic meaning is best accessed via subtle methods. The material accessed via surveys taps consciously available cognitions that do not necessarily play the major part in driving behaviour. In other words, when explicit questions are asked one taps reason-based explanations, attitudes and beliefs, which tend to be easily accessible but may hide not only the symbolic, but also the emotional and experiential material that drives cognition and behaviour.

What Kind of Research Questions is Thematic Analysis Most Suited to Addressing?

TA is best suited to elucidating the specific nature of a given group's conceptualization of the phenomenon under study. In my own work this has ranged from the public's conceptualizations of emerging infectious diseases (EID) such as AIDS (Joffe, 1999), the Ebola virus (Joffe & Haarhoff, 2002) and methicillin-resistant *Staphylococcus aureus* (MRSA; Joffe *et al.*, in press; Washer *et al.*, 2008), to mass media conceptualizations of these entities (e.g., Washer & Joffe, 2006). It has been used in the mental health arena in a similar way; for example, Morant's (2006) exploration of the social representations of mental illness from the perspective of French and British mental health practitioners. I use TA to discern possible identity issues associated with the representations of each disease and their impact on lay people's sense of personal and societal concern. More specifically, a key thread running through the EID findings is that there is a tendency to distance self and in-group from vulnerability to such diseases via a set of symbolic associations to marginalized, non-dominant groups and foreigners. The nuances of such associations are well tapped by TA, a method that can capture latent meaning while remaining systematic.

What Kinds of Data are Most Appropriate and From Whom Should They be Collected?

Verbal interview (or focus group) data or textual newspaper data tend to be at the root of thematic research. However, open-ended responses to questionnaire items, diaries, video material, images and essays can also be thematically analysed. Interview data are usually collected via semi-structured interviews: an interview with 5–7 topics that the respondent is prompted to talk about (see Wilkinson *et al.*, 2004). This imposes topic areas on people's thinking, where it may be preferable to gain a more naturalistic inroad into people's meaning systems concerning the phenomenon under study.

Instead of using topics introduced by the researchers as the basis for the interview, I have developed a more naturalistic method to elicit material. It produces data that follow the pathways of the respondent's thoughts and feelings rather than imposing questions and topic areas. To obtain these data the meeting with each respondent begins with a task that elicits first thoughts: respondents are presented with a grid containing four empty boxes. They are prompted to write or draw in each box any word, image or feeling that comes to mind concerning the research issue. Prior to this they are only given a very general sense of the field of study; for example, being invited to an interview on 'a public health issue' in the example in Box 15.1.

Box 15.1 Instruction Given to Elicit Free Associations

The following is an example of the instructions given for this grid method. The grid presented to respondents in a study of public engagement with MRSA in Britain was preceded by the following instruction 'We are interested in what you associate with MRSA. Please list the different images and words you associate with MRSA using these boxes. Include everything you associate with one image and/or word into one box' (Joffe *et al.*, in press; see also Solberg *et al.*, 2010).

Once first associations have been written or drawn, respondents are asked to talk about the content of each box in the order that the boxes have been completed. The aim is to elicit subjectively relevant material with a minimum of interference, to tap 'stored' naturalistic ways of thinking about a given topic and to then pursue the chains of association or pathways of thought that the respondents go down. Each interview is then transcribed and entered into a qualitative software package such ATLAS.ti, NUD*IST or NVivo.

In terms of who such data should be collected from, the decision concerning how many participants are required has vexed researchers who use TA. There is no notion of 'power' for the choice of the sample. A power analysis, for those working quantitatively, can be used to calculate the minimum sample size the researcher requires to accept the outcome of a statistical test with a particular level of confidence. The choice of sample size for a TA rests upon certain guiding principles: because the researcher is generally looking at group-based variation and/or similarity across groups, sufficient numbers of participants in each group are needed to make valid comparisons that are likely to reveal group-based threads in the data rather than idiosyncratic tangents of meaning. Furthermore, the sample size generally needs be divisible – for equal cell sizes to be used – so a primary number is not desirable. Because the idea is to look at patterning, sufficient numbers are required to discern patterns within the data set as a whole and across subgroups thereof. According to such criteria, numbers such as 32, 48, 60 and 80 are appropriate and when work is cross-cultural one multiplies these sample sizes by the number of cultures one is studying. These are large sample sizes in comparison to most qualitative approaches. However, large data sets can be handled with the aid of computer packages. Such packages also allow for systematic examination across the data at co-occurring themes, the sequence of themes and other more complex relations between themes, in a way that would be very difficult manually.

A more fundamental issue is what the accounts provided by a given sample represent. How do they relate to what a representative sample might have revealed about the topic? Each individual's account contains threads of the social thinking in which the individual is embedded. So, in individuals one picks up the thinking that surrounds them in their social environments, as well as the more idiosyncratic ways in which they position themselves in relation to this context. Using qualitative data sets to full advantage involves comparing the views and experiences of respondents who have been selected precisely – indeed, purposively – to illuminate potentially important differences and similarities. In other words, samples must be selected purposively in accordance with the research questions, to enhance how potential group differences and similarities, as well as intra-group variation, can be illuminated.

What Approach is Taken to the Involvement of Research Participants, Including Mental Health Service Users?

There has been a major expansion in service user involvement/user-led research in mental health over recent years. Qualitative research by service users often draws on generic thematic methods, rather than on TA per se. However, there is a growing body of research that uses TA. Gilburt *et al.*'s (2008) TA of service users' experiences of psychiatric hospital admission in the UK not only prioritizes the voice of users, but is led by two service user researchers.

A further cluster of studies using TA concern themselves with subjective experiences of different therapies, such as Allen *et al.*'s (2009) exploration of participants' subjective experience of Mindfulness-Based Cognitive Therapy for the treatment of their depression. TA analysis is also a powerful tool for casting light on non-use of mental health services. Its potential utility in this regard can be seen via a TA pertaining to the mental health and psychotherapy sphere (Johnston, 2000), which casts light on barriers to service use (Box 15.2).

Box 15.2 Some of the Findings From the TA on Non-use of Mental Health Services

The study explored the meanings people with no direct experience of psychological services assigned to the concept 'the psychologist' using aspects of the social representations framework and a TA. It showed that a sample of lower socioeconomic status Londoners, who had no contact with mental health services, represented the psychologist as a medical expert, in particular, of the mind. Furthermore, there was considerable consensus in linking the psychologist to strong emotional responses based on threat. The two were connected in that when confounded with the psychiatrist, the psychologist was seen to have the power to section people. Fear was also associated with other symbolizations of the psychologist: as akin to a mind-reader, parasite and archaeologist (as in excavating and 'digging up dirt'). Furthermore, fear sprang from the confounding of the 'sickness' of clients and that of the psychologist, as in 'one has to be a

(Continued)

Box 15.2 (*Cont'd*)

psycho to want to work with psychos'. Although a range of fears and stigma were pervasive, a model of the psychologist as helpful was also evident, particularly among females. The findings complement those from the existing survey-based help-seeking literature concerning treatment fearfulness, particularly among older people and men, but add insight into the symbolizations that form the barriers to help-seeking. A depth understanding of social representations of the psychologist can sensitize clinicians to the preconceptions that clients bring to the encounter. It can also aid efforts to promote psychological services by highlighting widely circulating representations that block the desire to seek help (adapted from Johnston, 2000).

How to Use This Method

There are surprisingly few published guides on to how to carry out TA, and it is often used in published studies without clear specification of the techniques employed. However, there are a few useful guides, including Boyatzis (1998), Braun and Clarke (2006) and Joffe and Yardley (2004). This chapter moves to laying out the set of key steps involved in a TA.

Examining the full data set as a precursor to developing a coding frame

Having read and re-read the entire corpus of data (or if images constitute one's data, had a careful look through all), one needs to create a conceptual tool with which to classify, understand and examine the data. Thus, one begins to devise a coding frame (also termed a 'coding manual' or 'coding book') to guide the TA. It contains the full set of codes that one chooses to apply to the data set. It is developed on the basis of both inductive codes grounded in the content of the data, and more theoretically driven codes inspired by past research in the area. Thus, in devising a coding frame for the TA of social representations of MRSA, Joffe *et al.* (in press)drew on social representational work on responses to other EIDs, the themes regarding MRSA found in national newspapers (Washer & Joffe, 2006) and an inductive reading of the full set of interviews. Table 15.1 is a small section of that coding frame.

For each code, its name appears in the first column, a definition of what should be classified with this code appears in the second, and an example of material that should be coded with this code appears in the third column. In both examples that appear in Table 15.1 one can see that the context is important. Such statements are made in the context of discussing the causes of MRSA in the interview. Furthermore, what one sees in these excerpts is that they contain other meanings too. So, for example, the 'cause–cleaners–foreign' is also coded 'cause–subcontracting of cleaning'. Multiple codes can be assigned to the same excerpt in a TA. Devising this frame is taxing and

Table 15.1 Section of the MRSA Coding Frame

Code-name	Definition	Example
META: CAUSES	**Explicit statement about the causes of MRSA**	
Cause–body products	Cause of MRSA is transmission of body products, such as sputum	'Not nice at all. I mean at the end of the day it's like when someone's lying in front of you who's sick as anything, he's coughing, he's puking, he's sneezing and you're sitting in the same environment, aren't you. You're sitting in the same room even though there's another 8 people with you, but this person's so bad he should, you know, common-sense, he should be on his own'
Cause–cleaners–foreign	Cause of MRSA is foreign cleaners	'It [cleaning] is subcontracted, outsourced, and the guy that's, that's looking after him is looking after 150 hospitals and this guy's being paid £1.50 an hour, illegal immigrant, so it's supervision again. Nobody cares'

time-consuming as there are no standardized categories to draw on; one devises a coding frame that will enable one to answer one's research question(s) in a balanced manner.

Checking the reliability of the coding frame

Once the codes have been developed, refined and clearly described in the coding frame, the researcher should determine its reliability. A rigorous way to ascertain reliability is to calculate the correspondence between the applications of the codes to the data by two independent coders. This should be applied to a substantial proportion of the data, usually 10–20%. In the study of public engagement with MRSA, having defined and operationalized what content was to be coded under each code, two researchers coded the same 20% of the data set independently. Rather than report the percentage of corresponding codes, in this case, where there was inconsistency, the relevant code was more carefully described and operationalized via a discussion between the two researchers. A new coding frame was then produced with more clearly and explicitly defined codes. The aim was to increase the transparency of the coding frame such that those using it would consistently apply the same codes to the same excerpts. In a more rigorous version of inter-rater reliability one reports the degree of concordance between coders. If it is high (e.g., above 75%) this coding frame is regarded as relatively transparent and reliable.

Coding the data using a computer-assisted data analysis package

Once a coding frame has been devised and reliability checked, the entire data set must be coded anew. Coding is the widely accepted term for categorizing data: taking chunks of text and labelling them as falling into certain categories, in a way that allows for later retrieval and analysis. Coding tells the researcher in how many interviews the category occurs and, if relevant, how many times it occurs within an interview. It also allows for analysis of the relationship of this code to other codes, in terms of co-occurrence and sequencing.

Because a rigorous TA must draw on a substantial number of interviews, computer-assisted data coding and analysis is most appropriate. Packages used for thematic analyses range from ATLAS.ti to NUD*IST to NVivo, among others. Computers cannot analyse textual data in the way that they can numerical data, yet, as a mechanical aid, the computer is able to enhance research for the following reasons: it allows researchers to deal with many more interviews than manual analyses can; because it can handle large data sets useful comparisons between groups can be made; the researcher is assisted in looking at patterns of codes, links between codes, sequencing and co-occurrence in a highly systematic fashion, because retrieval of data is made far easier.

Analysing the data using a data analysis package

When all of the data have been categorized, the analysis can begin. The analysis facilitates examination of the themes and their inter-connections, and the prevalence of the themes in the sample and subsamples. In a TA, especially one underpinned by a theory such as social representations, the nuances of the high frequency themes are explored in depth, as are group-based differences (such as those pertaining to gender, class or other groupings that emerge as relevant to answering the research question). The question arises concerning what to 'do with' idiosyncratic mentions of a particular theme. While idiosyncratic or occasional responses cannot, of course, be categorized as prevalent themes, they may nevertheless be important. For example, they may express what many in the sample take for granted, or articulate something that most members of the sample find difficult to voice.

Packages such as ATLAS.ti allow researchers to examine the patterning of themes across the range of interviews, and the common pathways or chains of association within interviews. More specifically, the filtering functions of such packages allow researchers to retrieve the patterns of codes prevalent in particular groups (e.g., different demographics), and such patterns can be retrieved as frequency charts, lists of textual excerpts, or visually, as visual networks. Box 15.3 contains an excerpt from the results section in the MRSA paper mentioned (Joffe et al., in press), showing how the most prevalent theme was presented. The paper began the reporting of the theme by presenting a typical excerpt that demonstrated the theme. Following this, the meanings and connections that constituted the theme were conveyed and also depicted in a chart that indicated the prevalence and links between the components of the theme visually. When the chart indicates 'better hygiene (n = 53)' as a way of countering MRSA, for example, this means that 53 of the 60 people in the sample specifically said that better hygiene would help to counter MRSA in some way.

Box 15.3 Presentation of Themes in a Results Section

Theme 1: Causal links made between dirt and MRSA

I just had this image of every hospital being disgustingly dirty and you're more likely to get ill, more ill than you were when you went in. So that's why [the first association in my grid is 'dirt']. So it was a bit of a worry. And I'm, I'm associating it with infection and germs and, you know, places that are not very clean. (38-year-old female, white British, broadsheet reader, hospitalized in the past year)

Almost all respondents represented MRSA via a framework (see Figure 15.1) that linked dirt to its cause. In particular, mention was made of MRSA being caused by the lack of hygiene within NHS hospitals, explained by deficits in handwashing practices and shortfalls in resources. In particular, staff supervision was regarded as deficient. Consequently, staff hygiene procedures were not enforced (also see structural theme 2).

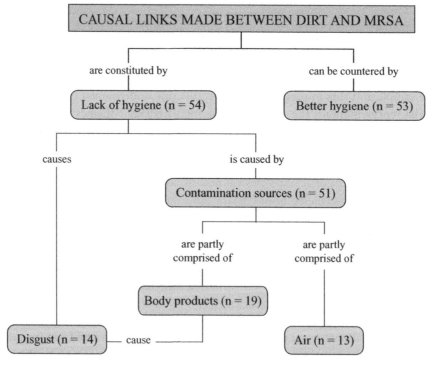

Figure 15.1 Causal links made between dirt and MRSA.

Also highly prevalent in the data concerning 'lack of hygiene' were mentions of a wide range of 'contamination sources' (Joffe et al., in press).

What Makes for a Better Quality Thematic Analysis?

In place of seeking accurate measurement of hypothetically related variables, and assessing their relationship statistically, good qualitative work seeks detailed complex interpretations of socially and historically located phenomena. It involves a shift from measurement to understanding; from causation to meaning; from statistical analysis to interpretation (Joffe, 2003; Smith *et al.*, 1995). A particular aspiration of TA is to balance being faithful to the data and being systematic in one's approach. What criteria can ensure that one does this?

A good TA must *describe the bulk of the data* – it must not simply select examples of text segments that support the arguments it wants to make. However, the prevalence of a given theme does not tell the whole story. The aspiration of TA is to reflect a balanced view of the data, and its meaning within a particular context of thoughts, rather than attaching too much importance to the frequency of codes abstracted from their context.

Science is concerned with how knowledge is produced. It is a systematic way of finding answers to research questions. An increasingly accepted view is that work becomes scientific by adopting methods of study *appropriate* to its subject matter (Silverman, 1993). Yet it also needs to produce knowledge systematically so that claims can be made concerning its *reliability* and *validity* (Silverman, 1993).

Beyond the aforementioned criteria that are conventionally associated with quantitative work, those using a TA need to *create a transparent trail* as to how they selected and collected their data, from whom and how it was analysed. This should involve providing access to the coding frame and if possible where the data is housed. In practice, this is often prohibited by ethical constraints (e.g., which state that one must destroy all of the interviews 6 months after the end of the study) and space constraints in journals (where the coding frame would occupy the valuable words of the word limit). Also in the name of transparency, researchers need to present systematically a sufficient portion of the original evidence in the written account to satisfy the sceptical reader of the relation between the interpretation and the evidence (Greenhalgh & Taylor, 1997). In practice, this too is often limited by space constraints in journals.

In addition to transparency, the following questions regarding the findings of a TA must be answered in the affirmative if the work is to be regarded as being of high quality. Are they *robust*, when compared with studies of similar topics using different methods and theoretical orientations? Do they incorporate the possibility of *revision*? Do they *expand current thinking*? Are they *useful* in advancing either theoretical knowledge or knowledge of the substantive issue under investigation? (see Silverman, 1993; Yardley, 2000).

What are the Recent Developments and Innovations Concerning this Method?

The most salient development regarding this method is the recent exponential growth in the use of TA as a method across a broad range of empirical papers. This includes a wide range of studies concerning mental and physical health, among many other areas. The citation of papers such as Braun and Clarke's (2006) step-by-step guide to conducting a TA, as well as growth in citation of Boyatzis' (1998) older book, reflects TA's increased use for empirical work both within psychology and beyond.

While TA is not intrinsically linked to a particular theory, it has been usefully paired with two in particular. A tradition is developing of pairing it with SRT (Moscovici & Duveen, 2000) to study how the public engage with a range of social issues (see e.g., Devine-Wright & Devine-Wright, 2009; Joffe, 1999; Joffe et al., in press). There is also a stream of studies using TA and SRT in relation to discerning media representations of a range of issues (see e.g., Joffe & Haarhoff, 2002; Smith & Joffe, 2009; Washer, 2004, 2006; Washer & Joffe, 2006; Washer et al., 2008).

Furthermore, TA's combination with phenomenology (e.g., Fereday & Muir-Cochrane, 2006), in its various forms, offers rich pickings for future work. Here the emphasis is on subjective experience and the 'taken-for-granted' of research participants. There is an emphasis on safeguarding the social reality of participants in a given study, rather than replacing it with a fictional reality that is the researcher's construct (Fereday & Muir-Cochrane, 2006). TA is well suited to this endeavour.

Conclusions

TA is an empirically driven approach for detecting the most salient patterns of content in interview, media and imagery content. It examines observable content as a first step in a more probing approach. A TA often does the following simultaneously: it looks at manifest themes as a route to understanding more latent, tacit content; its uses existing theoretical constructs to look at data while also allowing emerging themes to 'speak' by becoming the categories for analysis. Thus, pressing issues concerning the uptake of mental health services, or evaluation of the impacts of such services, can be explored systematically via TA.

Unlike many other qualitative methods, studies utilizing TA tend not to reflect on the impact of the researcher's preconceived ideas, and presence, on the data that emerge. This may, in part, be a residue from the aspects of the method that emerged from CA, with its more quantitative, apparently 'objective' epistemological positioning. While this may be seen as problematic, the emphasis on being systematic and transparent regarding the analysis (e.g., with a clearly laid out coding frame and reporting the outcome of reliability checks) allows other researchers to trace the process whereby the results were reached, and, if necessary, challenge them. In addition, as in all qualitative work, it is taken for granted that the interpretative aspects of TA are, by definition, influenced by the researcher's perspectives.

In terms of further developing this method, a fruitful future direction would be to return to a key aspect of the history of the field – Holton's development of the notion of 'themata' – to understand the tacit content that underpins the 'themes' in a TA.

Interestingly, a key figure within SRT, Marková (2007) links themata to the genesis of social representations and thus the link between TA, social representations and themata may provide fertile ground for further developing and deepening this burgeoning method.

Acknowledgements

I would like to thank Nicola Morant and the editors for useful improvement suggestions for this chapter. I would also like to acknowledge ERSC grant RES-000-22-1694 for development of the MRSA TA and EPSRC grant EP/F012179/1 for development of the Earthquake TA.

References

Allen, M., Bromley, A., Kuyken, W. & Sonnenberg, S.J. (2009). Participants' experiences of mindfulness-based cognitive therapy: 'It Changed Me in Just about Every Way Possible'. *Behavioural and Cognitive Psychotherapy*, 37, 413–430.

Boyatzis, R.E. (1998). *Transforming qualitative information: Thematic analysis and code development*. Thousand Oaks: Sage.

Braun, V. & Clarke, V. (2006). Using thematic analysis in psychology. *Qualitative Research in Psychology*, 3, 77–101.

Daly, J., Kellehear, A. & Gliksman, M. (1997). *The public health researcher: A methodological approach*. Melbourne, Australia: Oxford University Press.

Devine-Wright, H. & Devine-Wright, P. (2009). Social representations of electricity network technologies: Exploring processes of anchoring and objectification through the use of visual research methods. *British Journal of Social Psychology*, 48, 357–373.

Farr, R.M. & Moscovici, S. (2004). *Social representations*. Cambridge: Cambridge University Press.

Fereday, J. & Muir-Cochrane, E. (2006). Demonstrating rigor using thematic analysis: A hybrid approach of inductive and deductive coding and theme development. *International Journal of Qualitative Methods*, 5, 1–11.

Gilburt, H., Rose, D. & Slade, M. (2008). The importance of relationships in mental health care: A qualitative study of service users' experiences of psychiatric hospital admission in the UK. *BMC Health Services Research*, 8, 92.

Greenhalgh, T. & Taylor, R. (1997). How to read a paper: Papers that go beyond numbers (qualitative research). *British Medical Journal*, 315, 740–743.

Holloway, I. & Todres, L. (2003). The status of method: Flexibility, consistency and coherence. *Qualitative Research*, 3, 345–357.

Joffe, H. (1999) *Risk and 'the other'*. Cambridge: Cambridge University Press.

Joffe, H. (2003). Risk: from perception to social representation. *British Journal of Social Psychology*, 42 (1), 55–73.

Joffe, H. & Haarhoff, G. (2002) Representations of far-flung illnesses: The case of Ebola in Britain. *Social Science and Medicine*, 54, 955–969.

Joffe, H., Washer, P. & Solberg, C. (in press). Public engagement with emerging infectious disease: The case of MRSA in Britain. *Psychology and Health.*

Joffe, H. & Yardley, L (2004). Content and thematic analysis. In D. Marks & L. Yardley (Eds.) *Research methods for clinical and health psychology* (pp. 56–68). London: Sage.

Johnston, F. (2000). Social representation of psychology and the psychologist. Doctoral thesis, University College London, London.

Lupton, D. (1999). *Risk.* London and New York: Routledge.

Marková, I. (2007). Social identities and social representations: How are they related? In G. Moloney & I. Walker (Eds.) *Social representations and identity: Content, process, and power* (pp. 215–236). Hampshire: Palgrave Macmillan.

Merton, R.K. (1975). Thematic analysis in science: Notes on Holton's concept. *Science, 188,* 335–338.

Morant, N. (2006). Social representations and professional knowledge: The representation of mental illness among mental health practitioners. *British Journal of Social Psychology, 45,* 817–838.

Moscovici, S. & Duveen, G. (2000). *Social representations: Studies in social psychology.* Cambridge: Polity Press.

Silverman, D. (1993). *Doing qualitative research.* London: Sage.

Smith, C.P. (2000). Content analysis and narrative analysis. In H.T. Reis & C.M. Judd (Eds.) *Handbook of research methods in social and personality psychology* (pp. 313–335). New York: Cambridge University Press.

Smith, J.A., Harre, R. & Van Langenhove, L. (1995). *Rethinking methods in psychology.* London: Sage.

Smith, N. & Joffe, H. (2009). Climate change in the British Press: the role played by visual images. *Journal of Risk Research, 12,* 647–663.

Solberg, C., Rossetto, T. & Joffe, H. (2010). The social psychology of seismic hazard adjustment: Re-evaluating the international literature. *Natural Hazards and Earth Systems Sciences, 10,* 1663–1677.

Washer, P. (2004). Representations of SARS in the British newspapers. *Social Science and Medicine, 59* (12), 2561–2571.

Washer, P. (2006). Representations of mad cow disease. *Social Science and Medicine, 62,* 457–466.

Washer, P. & Joffe, H. (2006). The hospital 'superbug': Social representations of MRSA. *Social Science and Medicine, 63,* 2142–2152.

Washer, P., Joffe, H. & Solberg C. (2008). Audience readings of media messages about MRSA. *Journal of Hospital Infection, 70,* 42–47.

Wilkinson, S., Joffe, H. & Yardley, L. (2004). Qualitative data collection: interviews and focus groups. In D. Marks & L. Yardley (Eds.) *Research methods for clinical and health psychology* (pp. 39–55). London: Sage.

Willig, C. (in press). Perspectives on the Epistemological Bases for Qualitative Research. In H. Cooper (Ed.) *The handbook of research methods in psychology.* Washington, D.C.: American Psychological Association.

Yardley, L. (2000). Dilemmas in qualitative health research. *Psychology and Health, 15,* 215–228.

Further reading

Boyatzis, R.E. (1998). *Transforming qualitative information: Thematic analysis and code development.* London: Sage.

Braun, V. & Clarke, V. (2006). Using thematic analysis in psychology. *Qualitative Research in Psychology, 3,* 77–101.

Fereday, J. & Muir-Cochrane, E. (2006). Demonstrating rigor using thematic analysis: A hybrid approach of inductive and deductive coding and theme development. *International Journal of Qualitative Methods, 5,* 1–11.

Part III

Establishing Good Quality Qualitative Research in Mental Health

16

In Pursuit of Quality

Liz Spencer and Jane Ritchie

Deliberation on the meaning of quality in qualitative research has a long established pedigree but calls for systematic appraisal have intensified over the past two decades. Numerous quality checklists have been developed; indeed, both authors were involved in an initiative commissioned by the UK Cabinet Office (Spencer *et al.*, 2003). That project, together with the experience of teaching quality appraisal, confirmed the view that quality criteria should be viewed as part of an ongoing debate – and, if possible, should be framed as guidelines rather than prescriptive rules. Consequently, this chapter does not provide a quality framework as such, but it reviews some key concerns about quality in qualitative research and identifies some widely held *quality principles*. Each of these principles is examined in more detail through a set of *quality questions* that might be asked of a study and illustrated in relation to the qualitative methods discussed in this book.

The 'Quality' Debate

The debate in principle

The very idea of judging the quality of qualitative research is contested in the literature. Some objections are made on philosophical grounds. For example, Smith (1984, 1990) has argued that the *idealist* and *anti-foundational* nature of qualitative research makes it impossible to assess quality in the sense of applying a set of formalized criteria. Other writers, however, argue that qualitative research is not based on a single or shared set of philosophical assumptions and therefore the idea of judging quality cannot be simply dismissed on philosophical grounds (Altheide & Johnson, 1994; Hammersley, 1992; Phillips, 1990). Indeed, the methods described in this book make it clear that many

Qualitative Research Methods in Mental Health and Psychotherapy: A Guide for Students and Practitioners, First Edition.
Edited by D. Harper and A.R. Thompson.
© 2012 John Wiley & Sons, Ltd. Published 2012 by John Wiley & Sons, Ltd.

different ontological and epistemological positions are adopted by practising qualitative researchers.

Methodological concerns and objections are also raised. It is suggested that lack of methodological orthodoxy and the flexible nature of qualitative methods make them unsuitable for standardized assessment (Reicher, 2000; Schwandt, 1996). Some fear that too much emphasis on appraising methods, or 'methodolatry', could act as a straitjacket, limiting researchers' ability to innovate (Barbour, 2001; Chamberlain, 2000).

In part, concerns about the appraisal of qualitative research are responses to the idea of quality being assessed through the application of prescriptive rules or standards. However, if the concept of criteria is interpreted more loosely to mean guiding principles (Mason, 2002; Seale, 1999) or open-ended and evolving 'characterizing traits' that retain a role for individual judgement (Elliott *et al.*, 1999; Smith & Deemer, 2000), then some methodological and professional fears may be allayed.

The debate in practice

A key concern relates to whether or not quality involves the same constructs in qualitative and quantitative research. There is much disquiet about a simple transfer of accepted 'quantitative' criteria, given the wide range of epistemological and ontological positions adopted by qualitative researchers and the flexible non-standardized nature of their methods. Nevertheless, some argue for retaining concepts such as validity and reliability although the terms may be defined and applied in more or less traditional ways (Beck, 1993; Kirk & Miller, 1986; Le Compte & Goetz, 1982).

Guba and Lincoln have famously developed a parallel set of 'naturalistic' criteria to replace validity and reliability: *credibility, transferability, dependability* and *confirmability* (Guba & Lincoln 1981; Lincoln & Guba, 1985). Other researchers have retained the term validity, for example, but re-defined it to mean the impact of a study in promoting greater understanding or social change (Stiles, 1993). Finally, there are some who advocate abandoning all reference to notions of validity and reliability in favour of qualities such as intensive personal involvement, improvisation and flexibility (Agar, 1986).

Another major consideration is whether there are any generic qualitative indicators or whether each method requires its own criteria. While transparency about research decisions and analysis procedures might be accepted by some researchers as applicable across a number of different methods, more detailed aspects of quality may well be method-specific. For example, in conversation analysis, quality might be assessed in terms of the way a study makes evident the taken-for-granted competences people use in everyday conversations (see Chapter 13), whereas this would hold little relevance for an interview-based study. In document analysis, the question of whether or not an author directly witnessed an event might be seen as a way of establishing the 'authenticity' of a document (Platt, 1981), whereas treating a participant as a witness or informant in an interview-based study is only one of several different readings that can be made (Kvale & Brinkman, 2009).

Of course, questions about generic quality criteria – across different qualitative methods or even across qualitative and quantitative research – raise the issue of levels of specificity. At a very general level, some quality guidelines apply to both quantitative and qualitative research: appropriate methods, clarity of writing and contribution to knowledge have been cited as examples (Elliott *et al.*, 1999). Others might be intended specifically for qualitative research but apply to a range of different research methods, such as locating and understanding meanings in context. One way around this problem is to incorporate different levels into a quality framework, introducing core standards from which more specific criteria flow (Beck, 1993; Mays & Pope, 2000; Popay *et al.*, 1998).

A final practical concern relates to the kind of quality questions that should be asked and how they should be answered. Closed, yes/no questions are used in some quality frameworks whereas others adopt a more open-ended format. If an appraisal aims to be summative then there are problems about how to deal with studies where some aspects are deemed to have been well done but others not. Weighting and scoring various criteria may provide an overall assessment, but this approach is strongly resisted in some quarters of the qualitative research community.

Some Guiding Principles

Clearly, diverse positions are held on the desirability of evaluating qualitative research and, even when quality assessment is deemed possible, diverse appraisal criteria are suggested. However, it is possible to identify a number of recurring principles that underpin concepts of quality. These guiding principles, shared across many although not all epistemological perspectives, are described below, together with a series of questions that might be asked when appraising the quality of a qualitative study.

At the highest level of abstraction, quality principles concern assessments about the *contribution* of the research, the *credibility* it holds and the *rigour* of its conduct. However, because these might apply to any research, whatever its discipline or defining methodological paradigm, their meaning in qualitative research must be clarified.

Contribution

Contribution refers broadly to the value and relevance of research evidence. This may be to theory, to policy, to practice, to methodological development or to the lives and circumstances of individuals. Whatever the context, it requires an enhancement of existing understanding – or 'enlightenment'. With qualitative research, this contribution may be a case of providing an in-depth and nuanced understanding of the way particular people in particular circumstances construct, talk about or experience their micro-social world. It may identify processes, develop powerful analytical concepts or generate new hypotheses.

A key issue in debates about contribution concerns whether the findings of qualitative research can be said to have relevance beyond the participants or context of the study itself. In other words, is wider inference, external validity, transferability – however it may be termed – possible? There are very different views on the types of inference that can be drawn from qualitative research although some clear consensus that the basis of any generalization is quite distinct from that carried out in quantitative research, being based on assertional rather than probabilistic logic (Kvale, 1996; Stake, 2000).

One school of thought suggests that qualitative research can offer *inferential* generalization by which findings from one setting can be generalized to other settings or contexts (Lincoln & Guba, 1985). There are then those who believe that qualitative data can provide analytic or *theoretical* generalizations either through generating analytical concepts that can be applied more widely (Strauss & Corbin, 1998) or from case to theory through the application of analytical concepts or theoretical ideas (Seale, 1999). There are also those who would argue that qualitative research can be used for *representational* generalization by which findings can be inferred at a conceptual level from the study population to the parent population from which it was selected (Lewis & Ritchie, 2003).

Some writers, particularly those from post-modern schools of thought, would argue that wider inference is beyond the scope of qualitative research. There are no overarching meanings to be found because they are context specific, a product of time and space (Schwandt, 1997). Others judge the main contribution of a study in terms of its educative or emancipatory impact on participants rather than any inferential outcomes (Roman & Apple, 1990).

Credibility

Credibility relates to the defensibility and plausibility of claims made by research. It concerns not only the 'believability' of findings but also the ability to see how claims or conclusions have been reached. It raises a number of issues that lie at the heart of assessments of quality.

One of the most recurrent concerns the notion of *validity*, in particular its meaning and its relevance for qualitative research. Hammersley (1991), for example, has suggested that the traditional 'scientific' notion of internal validity (Cook & Campbell, 1979) was used to refer to whether or not an instrument was valid and measured what it purported to measure, and whether or not a particular measurement was valid or accurate. These twin concerns about methodological and interpretive validity have subsequently been adapted by researchers to fit their understanding of qualitative research. Methodological validity has been transposed to concerns about rigour, which can be demonstrated through careful documentation of the research process, as discussed below. Interpretive validity, on the other hand, is taken to refer to the adequacy of representation and to how convincingly a claim is made and backed up by evidence (Seale, 2007; Whittemore *et al.*, 2001).

If credibility rests on the evidence presented, then a key question concerns the nature of evidence in qualitative research. There are many possibilities including:

- Descriptive accounts portraying the composition and categorization of the raw data.
- Interpretative accounts showing how the data have been put together to develop explanations, reach conclusions and generate hypotheses or theories.

- Constructed representations such as diagrams, figures, case studies, and so on.
- Extracts of raw data.

It is generally agreed that some display of raw data should be included although views differ on the purpose this serves. Some writers argue that the original material is essential as part of the 'evidence' required – particularly in conversation or discourse analysis – others see it as amplificatory or illustrative to analytic representations.

There is also some consensus about the importance of defending claims through explicit demonstrations that negative cases have been examined or alternative explanations sought (Miles & Huberman, 1994; Potter, 1996; Seale, 1999; Silverman, 2000). *Validation* of research findings is also discussed in terms of triangulation, a process involving the use of different methods, sources or 'readings' to check the integrity of, or extend, inferences drawn from the data. But many writers argue that triangulation is better viewed as a way of honing a more sophisticated account than of validating a claim (Greene, 1994; Patton, 2002). Other approaches to validation include peer review (Hammersley, 1992), member validation (Angen, 2000; Stiles, 1993) and constant comparison methods (Adler & Adler, 1994; Gliner, 1994; Potter, 1996).

Rigour

Rigour may seem a somewhat incongruous word in the vocabulary of qualitative research, given its interactive, exploratory and interpretative nature. But, as was discussed above, rigour is seen as synonymous with methodological validity, which raises a host of issues concerned with the appropriateness of research decisions, the dependability of evidence and the general safe conduct of research.

The concept of *reliability* is considered particularly difficult in the context of qualitative research. If reliability is taken to mean *replication*, then the concept is often rejected because qualitative research uses flexible rather than standardized designs or methods. Reliability is sometimes discussed in terms of *consistency*; for example, would different researchers identify the same concepts or categories (Le Compte & Goetz, 1982), or would different researchers assign instances to the same concept or category (Ambert *et al.*, 1995; Armstrong *et al.*, 1997; Silverman, 2000)? However, the idea that consistency is possible does not fit well with all approaches. Indeed, many qualitative researchers would expect there to be some differences between the findings of different researchers. Consequently, some have proposed that reliability should be viewed in terms of *auditability*, *dependability* or *reflexivity* as discussed below.

The need for *objectivity* is often seen as an essential requirement of research but again this is problematic for qualitative inquiry. One response, which has been highlighted in feminist methodologies, is to consider any notion of neutrality as misguided because of the intricate relationship that will inevitably exist between the researcher and the researched (Bowles & Klein, 1983; Roberts, 1981). Seale (1999) argues that objectivity is an attitude of mind and requires researchers to stand back as far as possible in terms of their own values. A more common viewpoint, however, is a call for *reflexivity* through which researchers not only describe the research process, but also assess the impact of their role and presence, and declare the values and theoretical orientation that have guided their research.

Careful documenting and reporting of research decisions, orientations, roles and impacts is often referred to in the literature as *auditability* or the *audit trail* (Lincoln & Guba, 1985; Merrick, 1999). A detailed audit, including fieldwork documents and analytical schema, usually only appears with a full account of the study's findings (see e.g., Spencer & Pahl, 2006) although key features, such as the researcher's guiding values or the researcher–participant relationship are needed in articles, presentations or even summaries as a context to the research evidence.

The *defensibility* of approach and design is also seen to form part of well-constructed research. Of particular importance here are: a clear logic of inquiry, enabling the study to meet its aims (Fournier & Smith, 1993); a convincing rationale for the choice of method (Mason, 2002; Patton, 2002); and appropriate decisions surrounding the composition of the sample so that key research questions can be addressed (Mitchell & Bernaurer, 1998; Strauss & Corbin, 1998).

As may be apparent, through all the aspects of rigour described there are overarching requirements for appropriate decision making and thoroughness of conduct. What this entails in practice is examined and illustrated in the next section.

Quality in Practice

As will be evident from the preceding discussion, many different questions might be asked of a research study to assess its quality, depending on the philosophical and methodological stances that underpin the inquiry. It is therefore only feasible here to present a brief schema of elements that might be considered under the three guiding principles of contribution (Table 16.1), credibility (Table 16.2) and rigour (Table 16.3), and to illustrate some of these elements in more detail by reference to issues raised or studies described in earlier chapters. It must be stressed, however, that the purpose of the discussion is to offer examples rather than to provide an exhaustive or prescriptive set of criteria.

The form and extent of appraisal will clearly depend on what is being assessed at which stage of the research process. In a full account of a study, such as a book or a thesis, an appraiser would expect to see a wide range of quality questions addressed, including a detailed audit trail. With journal articles space will limit what can be included. Nevertheless, key aspects of the study should be displayed such as how, why and with what restrictions study participants were selected, how data collection or generation was carried out and some insights into how the analysis was conducted. On the latter point, for example, it is all too often the case that authors support their findings only with extracts of raw data without illustrating how their analytic output was constructed. For research proposals assessors will want to see clear rationales for the choice of methods and how these relate to the aims of the study. Again analysis is often a weak point here – a statement that a particular approach or software package will be used tells a reviewer little about the analytical process that will be followed.

Table 16.1 Contribution: The extent to which the study has contributed to wider knowledge and understanding or had some utility within the original context

Central questions	Quality questions relate to	Illustration
How has knowledge/ understanding been extended?	• In what ways the study aimed to contribute to knowledge or help bring change; how well it achieved this • Clarity of discussion on how findings have brought new insights/alternative ways of thinking • Discussion of how hypotheses/propositions/findings relate to pre-existing knowledge; consideration of rival explanations or theories • Discussion of limitations of evidence and what remains unknown or unclear	The study described in Chapter 9 used existential-informed hermeneutic phenomenology to explore spirituality and meaning-making at the end of life. Two modes of being were identified: 'everyday' and 'transcendent'. A quality appraiser might look for an account of the way the finding relates to other evidence of the experience of spirituality at the end of life or spirituality in other contexts
How well is the basis of drawing wider inference explained?	• Discussion of whether and how findings/conclusions extend beyond the contexts of the study • Nature and adequacy of evidence supplied to support claims for wider inference or transferability • Level of description of the contexts in which study is set to allow assessment of applicability to other settings • Discussion of limitations to drawing inference beyond study contexts or participants	In grounded theory and IPA, wider inference is drawn from a population to a sample. With thematic analysis (see Chapter 15), it is suggested that elements of broader social thinking are contained in individual accounts. Conversation analysts (see Chapter 13) look for properties of the whole that are present in individual cases rather than at the aggregate level. In quality appraisal, one might look to see if properties identified in one study are compared with those found in another in order to ascertain the contribution of a particular piece of research
What value has the study evidence had for participants/ service users?	• Discussion of how study was intended to contribute to the lives, circumstances or treatments of participants/service users and whether/how it has done so • Discussion of ways in which roles or status of study participants/service users have been enhanced or affected by the study	In Chapter 12 it is argued that narrative analysis can be liberating for participants and an appraiser might look for a description of this empowerment process in a particular study

Table 16.2 Credibility: The extent to which findings are believable and well-founded

Central questions	Quality questions relate to	Illustration
How does the evidence support the findings?	• The way in which the evidence provides clear links between the findings and the data *Descriptive findings* • Discussion of the way perceptions and experiences vary in relation to key themes and concepts • Demonstration of the way higher order categories, groupings, classifications and typologies fit the data: whether there are any outlier or negative cases (in cross-sectional analysis) *Explanations* • Discussion of what is being explained (linkage, behaviour, a particular outcome) and whether the explanation is implicit (given by participants themselves) or implicit (inferred by the researcher) • Discussion of the way pieces of evidence fit together to underpin the argument, and whether alternative explanations have been tried	Several contributors to this book advocate the inclusion of data extracts or verbatim quotations to back up claims and show a sceptical reader how interpretation is rooted in the data (see e.g., Chapters 11 and 15) Taking account of negative or deviant cases is raised as an important aspect of grounded theory (see Chapter 10), discourse analysis (see Chapter 11) conversation analysis (see Chapter 13) and thematic analysis (see Chapter 15). An appraiser might search for ways in which these have been explored; for example, to extend a hypothesis or show the boundaries of inclusion within a typology or a theory

| How plausible are the findings? | • Discussion of the way in which findings fit with existing knowledge
• Demonstration of a persuasive argument if findings are not initially plausible | Plausibility is not explicitly raised in the different methods chapters but is implicit in authors' discussions of the need for clear, transparent and reflexive documentation of the research process. Providing a detailed audit trail makes it possible for readers to assess credibility when plausibility is not immediately obvious (see below) |
| What forms of validation been attempted? Why? Why not? | • Discussion of any validation efforts in terms of triangulation, member validation, peer review and how these have led to a refinement of the conclusions | In Chapter 6 the author recommends that one or more credibility checks be included, such as auditing the analysis process, using multiple analysts or asking for participants' confirmation or comment. However, member/participant validation is not necessarily appropriate for all qualitative methods (see Chapters 9 and 11). While descriptive accounts can be strengthened in this way, the technical language used in more interpretive accounts may not be accessible to research participants. An appraiser might assess the rationale for a particular validation strategy being adopted and the way in which it enhanced the credibility of the study findings |

Table 16.3 Rigour: The transparency of the research process, the defensibility of design decisions and the thoroughness of conduct

Central questions	Quality questions relate to	Illustration
How well-documented and reflexive is the research process?	• Clarity about the values and assumptions that guided the research • Description of how and why key decisions were made/actions were taken at each stage of the research process • Inclusion of/reference to key documents (e.g., letters to participants, consent forms, topic guides, analytic frameworks) • Discussion of field relationships, stance adopted by the researcher and the impact of research on participants	The importance of transparency and reflexivity is highlighted in a number of different chapters. Suggestions include documenting all stages of the research process (see Chapter 8) and memo-writing in which the researcher keeps track of his or her analytical journey (see Chapter 10). In the study described in Chapter 9, a researcher used a diary to document the possible impact of her own good health on what terminally ill participants told her and her reactions to findings that challenged her initial preconceptions. An appraiser would welcome this kind of reflexivity being referenced in a report, either as part of the methods discussion or in a technical appendix. Despite the importance attached to reflexivity in qualitative research, reflexive accounts are not routinely included
How well defended is the overall research strategy and design?	• Description of rationale for qualitative research or the contribution of a qualitative component in mixed methods designs: how and why qualitative research is appropriate for the field or research aims/question(s) • Clear account of the appropriateness of the research strategy chosen (e.g., theory-led or exploratory/single stage or longitudinal)	Inductive qualitative methods, such as grounded theory, are seen as well-suited to a broad range of open-ended research questions that focus on meanings, experiences and processes (see Chapter 10). The authors argue – as should researchers providing a rationale for their choice of qualitative methods – that an inductive approach is particularly appropriate in the field of clinical psychology because it explores the subjective experience of 'marginalized' or 'stigmatized' people. An appraiser might want to know if other designs were considered and why they were rejected

How appropriate are the methods used?	• Description of rationale for use of methods chosen; how they link to study objectives; how they relate to nature and circumstances of the study population • Consideration of other methods and why rejected • Limitations of methods used and implications	In Chapter 12, the authors maintain that narrative analysis is a particularly appropriate research method for studying the experience of health service users. Describing a study of men who had suffered serious injuries that prevented them form working full-time, they argue that – by telling their own stories – participants were able to locate their experiences within a broader life history perspective in contrast to the more limited way they were perceived by agency staff. An appraiser would look for this kind of confirmation that the choice of methods was justified
Have well have ethical issues been considered and addressed?	• Evidence of sensitivity to research contexts and study participants • Discussion of way research was presented to participants, consent negotiated and anonymity/confidentiality protected • Need for measures to provide information, advice or services to study participants and how met • Discussion of any negative impacts of participation and how dealt with	Qualitative researchers who are also clinical psychologists face difficult ethical challenges (see Chapter 3). Confidentiality, privacy, informed consent, harm and power are particularly complex because of the interaction between participant and researcher, the way qualitative interviews can cover unanticipated ground, and the dual role of researcher and clinician. Examples are given of actions taken in a number of studies: requesting participants' consent for particular excerpts and quotes to be reported; separating researcher and clinician roles by drawing boundaries in the interview so that clinical matters are addressed afterwards or by prioritizing the clinical role and excluding a participant from the study. Including information about such courses of action would be welcomed by a quality appraiser

(continued)

Table 16.3 *(Continued)*

Central questions	Quality questions relate to	Illustration
How well defended is the sample design/target selection of participants, cases or documents?	• Description of study locations/ areas and how and why chosen • Rationale for inclusion of selected participants/documents/ settings • Discussion of characteristics and circumstances of study participants; how these relate to wider population from which they come; extent to which saturation achieved • Discussion of missing coverage in achieved participation and implications for study evidence	Several authors refer to the small sample sizes used in qualitative research. However, sample composition is of more relevance than sample size. A purposive sample, the composition of which gives appropriate coverage and permits desired comparisons to be made is advocated in a number of chapters. An appraiser would look for a detailed and convincing rationale, linking the sample design to the research questions or aims. For some qualitative methods, appraisers might also look for some comparison between the study group and the population from which it was drawn to see what characteristics or circumstances are covered or missing
How well was the data generation process carried out?	• Description of how and by whom data generation was carried out and any difficulties encountered • Description of methods of recording spoken data (whether generated or naturally occurring) and any restrictions this imposed • Description of conventions for taking field notes • Demonstration through portrayal and use of data that depth, detail, richness and nuance have been achieved	The hallmarks of good quality data generation and collection vary across different qualitative methods. Narrative analysts should take care not to interrupt the narrative flow during an interview, but leave the participant free to tell his or her own story (see Chapter 12). Thematic analysts might capture participants' spontaneous thoughts, images or feelings, rather than introducing predefined topics (see Chapter 15). In conversation analysis, based on naturally occurring conversations rather than interview data, there are widely accepted guidelines for transcription so that features of the interaction, such as hesitation, are captured

| How thoroughly was the analysis carried out? | • Discussion of the analysis process adopted and the extent to which all data have been reviewed
• Discussion of the way analytical themes and concepts were developed and how well they fit the data
• The retention of complexity, variation and nuance despite the need for data reduction and synthesis
• Evidence of attention to outliers and negative cases
• The inclusion of participants' terms and understandings
• Demonstration that the analysis takes account of and preserves the context of the data | In Chapter 6 the author recommends that themes/categories should be grounded in the data, with one or two examples provided for the main categories. Detailed illustrations of the analysis process, the application of codes and the development of more interpretive themes are given in relation to a number of different methods (see, e.g., Chapters 8, 12, 13 and 15). For any given study, appraisers would want to see worked examples such as these included in thematic chapters or in a methodological appendix |
| How clear and coherent is the reporting? | • How well the structure of the document is set out and signposted
• How well the findings relate to the original aims and objectives or any divergence from these is explained
• The interweaving of interpretation and evidence; the use of examples to illustrate key themes or arguments and convey the richness of the data
• Accessibility of information for target audiences
• Clarity of narrative, story or constructed thematic account | Several authors stress the importance of illustrating analytical themes and findings with examples and extracts of raw data. Including a clear audit trail of research decisions is also advocated in many of the chapters. For applied research, appraisers will also be concerned with the accessibility of the reporting for the target audiences expected |

Conclusions

The call for criteria by which qualitative research can be assessed has grown significantly in the last two decades. Many guidelines and frameworks for quality appraisal have been developed across a range of policy-related fields and academic disciplines, but the question of whether and how qualitative research can be formally assessed remains the subject of much debate.

There is nevertheless some agreement on two issues. First, there are some widely held central principles of good practice that can guide assessment. Secondly, any assessment of quality will need to be tuned to the philosophical and methodological base of a specific study.

The quality principles and questions identified in this chapter are offered as examples of issues that might be considered. However, it is important to emphasize that the quality of any particular research study will – in large part – be a product of the proficiency, experience and creativity of the research team. Assessing that quality will always involve professional judgement.

References

Adler, P.A. & Adler, P. (1994). Observational techniques. In N.K. Denzin & Y.S. Lincoln (Eds.) *Handbook of qualitative research* (pp. 377–392). Thousand Oaks, CA: Sage.

Agar, N.H. (1986). *Speaking of ethnography: Qualitative research methods series, no 2.* London: Sage.

Altheide, D.L. & Johnson, J.M. (1994). Criteria for assessing interpretive validity. In N.K. Denzin & Y.S. Lincoln (Eds.) *Handbook of qualitative research* (pp. 485–499). Thousand Oaks, CA: Sage.

Ambert, A., Adler, A., Adler, P. & Detzner, D.F. (1995). Understanding and evaluating qualitative research. *Journal of Marriage and the Family, 57,* 879–893.

Angen, M.J. (2000). Evaluating interpretive inquiry: Reviewing the validity debate and opening the dialogue. *Qualitative Health Research, 10,* 378–395.

Armstrong, D., Gosling, A., Weinman, J. & Marteau, T. (1997). The place of inter-rater reliability in qualitative research: An empirical study. *Sociology, 31,* 597–606.

Barbour, R.S. (2001). Checklists for improving rigour in qualitative research: A case of the tail wagging the dog? *British Medical Journal, 322,* 1115–1117.

Beck, C.T. (1993). Qualitative research: The evaluation of its credibility, fittingness and auditability. *Western Journal of Nursing Research, 15,* 263–266.

Bowles, G. & Klein, R.D. (1983). *Theories of women's studies.* Boston: Routledge and Kegan Paul.

Chamberlain, K. (2000). Methodolatry and qualitative health research. *Journal of Health Psychology, 5,* 285–296.

Cook, T. & Campbell, D. (1979). *Quasi experimentation.* Chicago: Rand McNally.

Elliott, R., Fischer, C.T. & Rennie, D.L (1999). Evolving guidelines for publication of qualitative research studies in psychology and related fields. *British Journal of Clinical Psychology, 38,* 215–229.

Fournier, D.M. & Smith, N.L. (1993). Clarifying the merits of argument in evaluation practice. *Evaluation and Programme Planning, 16,* 315–323.

Gliner, J.A. (1994). Reviewing qualitative research: Proposed criteria for fairness and rigor. *Occupational Therapy Journal of Research, 14*, 78–90.

Greene, J. (1994). Qualitative program evaluation: Practice and promise. In N.K. Denzin & Y.S. Lincoln (Eds.) *Handbook of qualitative research* (pp. 530–544). Thousand Oaks, CA: Sage.

Guba, E. & Lincoln, Y. (1981). *Effective evaluation.* San Francisco, CA: Jossey-Bass.

Hammersley, M. (1991). A note on Campbell's distinction between external and internal validity. *Quality and Quantity, 25*, 381–387.

Hammersley, M. (1992). *What's wrong with ethnography?* London: Routledge.

Kirk, J. & Miller, M. (1986). *Reliability and validity in qualitative research.* Newbury Park, CA: Sage.

Kvale, S. (1996). *InterViews: An introduction to qualitative research interviewing.* Thousand Oaks, CA: Sage.

Kvale, S. & Brinkmann, J. (2009). *InterViews: Learning the craft of qualitative research interviewing.* Thousand Oaks: Sage.

Le Compte, M. & Goetz, J. (1982). Problems of reliability and validity in ethnographic research. *Review of Educational Research, 52*, 31–60.

Lewis, J. & Ritchie, J. (2003). Generalising from qualitative research. In J. Ritchie & J. Lewis (Eds.) *Qualitative research practice* (pp. 263–286). London: Sage.

Lincoln, Y. & Guba, E. (1985). *Naturalistic inquiry.* Beverly Hills: Sage.

Mason, J. (2002). *Qualitative researching.* London: Sage.

Mays, N. & Pope, C. (2000). Quality in qualitative health research. In C. Pope & N. Mays (Eds.) *Qualitative research in health care* (pp. 89–102). London: BMJ Books.

Merrick, E. (1999). An exploration of quality in qualitative research: Are 'Reliability' and 'validity' relevant? In M. Kopala & L.A. Suzuki (Eds.) *Using qualitative methods in psychology* (pp. 25–36). Thousand Oaks, CA: Sage.

Miles, M.B. & Huberman, A.M. (1994). *Qualitative data analysis: An expanded sourcebook.* London: Sage.

Mitchell, R. & Bernauer, T. (1998). Empirical research on international environmental policy: Designing qualitative case studies. *Journal of Environment and Development, 7*, 4–31.

Patton, M.Q. (2002). *Qualitative research and evaluation methods.* Thousand Oaks, CA: Sage.

Phillips, D. (1990). Post-positivistic science myths and realities. In E. Guba (Ed.) *The paradigm dialogue* (pp. 31–45). Newbury Park, CA: Sage.

Platt, J. (1981). Evidence and proof in documentary research. 1: Some specific problems of documentary research. *Sociological Review, 29*, 31–52.

Popay, J., Rogers, A. & Williams, G. (1998). Rationale and standards for the systematic review of qualitative literature in health services research. *Qualitative Health Research, 8*, 341–351.

Potter, J. (1996). Discourse analysis and constructionist approaches: Theoretical background. In J.T.E. Richardson (Ed.) *Handbook of qualitative research methods for psychology and the social science* (pp. 125–140). Leicester: BPS Books.

Reicher, S. (2000). Against methodolatry: Some comments on Elliott, Fischer and Rennie. *British Journal of Clinical Psychology, 39*, 1–6.

Roberts, H. (1981). *Doing feminist research.* London: Sage.

Roman, L. & Apple, M. (1990.) Is naturalism a move away from positivism? Materialist and feminist approaches to subjectivity in ethnographic research. In E. Eisner & A. Peshkin (Eds.) *Qualitative inquiry in education: The continuing debate* (pp. 38–73). New York: Teachers College Press.

Schwandt, T.A. (1996). Farewell to criteriology. *Qualitative Inquiry, 2*, 58–72.

Schwandt, T.A. (1997). *Qualitative inquiry: A dictionary of terms.* Thousand Oaks, CA: Sage.

Seale, C. (1999). *The quality of qualitative research.* London: Sage.

Seale, C. (2007). Quality in qualitative research. In C. Seale, G. Gobo, J. Gubrium & D. Silverman (Eds.) *Qualitative research practice* (pp. 409–419). London: Sage.

Silverman, D. (2000). *Doing qualitative research: A practical handbook.* London: Sage.

Smith, J.K. (1984). The problem of criteria for judging interpretive inquiry. *Educational Evaluation and Policy Analysis, 6,* 397–391.

Smith, J.K. (1990). Goodness criteria: Alternative research paradigms and the problem of criteria. In E.G. Guba (Ed.) *The paradigm dialogue* (pp. 167–187). London: Sage.

Smith, J.K. & Deemer, D. (2000). The problem of criteria in the age of relativism. In N. Denzin & Y. Lincoln (Eds.) *Handbook of qualitative research* (3rd edn, pp. 915–932). Thousand Oaks, CA: Sage.

Spencer. L. & Pahl, R.E. (2006). *Rethinking friendship: Hidden solidarities today.* Princeton: Princeton University Press.

Spencer, L., Ritchie, J., Lewis, J. & Dillon, L. (2003). *Quality in qualitative evaluation: A framework for assessing research evidence.* London: Government Chief Social Researcher's Office.

Stake, R. (2000). Case studies. In N.K. Denzin & Y.S. Lincoln (Eds.) *Handbook of qualitative research* (pp. 435–454). Thousand Oaks, CA: Sage

Stiles, W.B. (1993). Quality control in qualitative research. *Clinical Psychology Review, 13,* 593–618.

Strauss, A.L. & Corbin, J. (1998). *Basics of qualitative research: Grounded theory procedures and techniques.* Thousand Oaks, CA: Sage.

Whittemore, R., Chase, S.K. & Mandle, C.L. (2001). Validity in qualitative research. *Qualitative Health Research, 11,* 522–537.

Further reading

Barbour, R.S. (2001). Checklists for improving rigour in qualitative research: A case of the tail wagging the dog? *British Medical Journal, 322,* 1115–1117.

Elliott, R., Fischer, C.T. & Rennie, D.L (1999). Evolving guidelines for publication of qualitative research studies in psychology and related fields. *British Journal of Clinical Psychology, 38,* 215–229.

Spencer, L., Ritchie, J., Lewis, J. & Dillon, L. (2003). *Quality in qualitative evaluation: A framework for assessing research evidence.* London: Government Chief Social Researcher's Office.

17

Emerging Issues and Future Directions

David Harper and Andrew R. Thompson

In this book we have gathered together a range of contributors who have provided short and accessible introductions to either a key theme in qualitative research or a particular research method. The chapters devoted to particular methods of analysis have followed a similar structure so that readers can compare the way each addresses important issues and judge whether that will be the method most suited to addressing their research questions.

In this chapter, we would like to discuss some of the cross-cutting themes emerging from the rest of the book. We will look, in turn, at the range of data available for qualitative research, emerging ethical issues, service user involvement, evidence-based practice and dissemination. Finally, we will consider the future directions that qualitative research in mental health and psychotherapy might take.

The Range of Data Available for Qualitative Research

One of our intentions in including two chapters on data collection in qualitative research was to demonstrate the wide array of methods available. Our experience as teachers, supervisors and examiners is that the semi-structured interview has become as ubiquitous in qualitative research theses by trainee mental health professionals as the questionnaire is in quantitative research. Interviews are an important – but not the only – data collection technique. Indeed, in some instances they may be inappropriate, because they are only a proxy – and sometimes a misleading proxy – for the kinds of things in which the investigator is interested. Chapter 5 identified some of the alternatives to interviews which are available whilst Chapter 6 provided suggestions of data collection methods suited to the exploration of change processes within psychotherapy.

Qualitative Research Methods in Mental Health and Psychotherapy: A Guide for Students and Practitioners, First Edition.
Edited by D. Harper and A.R. Thompson.
© 2012 John Wiley & Sons, Ltd. Published 2012 by John Wiley & Sons, Ltd.

Given that much qualitative research uses verbal data, there is a particular issue in conducting research with participants from diverse cultural backgrounds. Some qualitative researchers avoid recruiting participants who are not able to converse well in English. Whilst this may be done for understandable reasons (e.g., to aim for a more homogeneous sample or because funds are not available for interpreters), this leads to the ethical problem that such groups become systematically excluded (Nimisha Patel, personal communication). This is an issue with which a number of learned societies have been grappling over recent years (Salway *et al.*, 2009).

Many mental health practitioners and psychotherapists will already be familiar with some of the complexities of working with interpreters in their everyday work and there are a number of helpful texts available for guidance (e.g., Shackman, 1985; Tribe & Raval, 2003). A number of practitioner organizations have also published good practice guidance. An increasing number of qualitative researchers are seeking to work alongside interpreters. However, interpreters do exactly that – they *interpret* rather than necessarily providing a word-for-word translation. As a result there are difficult choices to be made: is conceptual clarity more important than verbatim translation? Analysis here requires close attention to nuance and context. There needs to be open discussion between the researcher and interpreter about the aims of the study early in the research design process and funding may need to be sought.

One could make a case that, for methods with a focus on the way in which language is used (e.g., Discourse Analysis), research on non-English speaking participants is best conducted by researchers who are also fluent speakers of that language (see e.g., Vara & Patel, in press). However, where the focus is not on language use per se then interpreted speech could be included, using techniques such as back-translation and feedback from participants. In relation to Interpretative Phenomenological Analysis (IPA), for example, Smith (2004) suggests that researchers should conduct a cost–benefit analysis on a case-by-case basis.

Emerging Ethical Issues

As Chapter 3 demonstrated, there are a number of complex ethical issues specific to qualitative research. Indeed, as qualitative approaches develop and topics evolve, new ethical challenges may present themselves. One that often is not discussed in much detail is that, because more detail is given about participants, it renders them potentially more identifiable. For this reason it is good practice to think carefully about what readers need to know about your participants in order to have a context for your findings. There are a range of possibilities here. For example, some researchers suggest reporting some demographic information (e.g., ethnicity in areas where there are not large numbers of people from different ethnic backgrounds) in group terms rather than providing a table of participants where all the details are listed for each participant because this can make people identifiable. Some researchers and practitioners may feel that important contextual information is lost but, even so, when providing a table some information can be provided in a way that is less identifying (e.g., an age range rather than an exact age, a professional grouping rather than exact job title, etc.). However, in cases of a rare or easily identifiable group of some kind, total anonymity may not be possible and so it is best to be clear about this with participants and ask them what they are happy to disclose. Indeed, Parker (2005) has argued that, in certain cases, it may be more ethical not to promise anonymity.

Another emerging issue relates to recruitment. In Chapter 3, Andrew Thompson and Eleni Chambers discussed some of the more paternalistic assumptions of some ethics committees. This can cause a problem when trying to recruit participants who may be hard to access and who may not participate if there are too many hurdles placed in their way – for example, homeless people who may not be continuously engaged with mental health services. However, a rationale can sometimes be made for procedures where participants opt out rather than opt in in order to avoid inadvertently excluding groups of potential participants.

Of course, ethical issues can arise not only in relation to procedural aspects, but also the interpretations researchers place on participants' words (Harper, 2003), the implications they draw from their studies and the way in which these implications may be understood by service users, policy makers and the wider public when researchers, understandably, wish to move from a descriptive mode (in relation to their study) to a prescriptive one (in relation to mental health theory or policy). For example, within qualitative research there is a debate about the notion of coherence in relation to narratives. Gergen (1994) has noted that coherent narratives tend to be viewed as inherently more plausible. However, this descriptive account can then be interpreted by policy makers as making the normative claim that narratives that are not coherent are less plausible. Indeed, the UK Home Office (responsible for immigration, refugees and claims for political asylum) uses the coherence of a refugee's account as proxy evidence of its plausibility. However, there is increasing evidence that traumatic experiences can lead to fragmented memories and narratives (Herlihy et al., 2002; Hyvärinen et al., 2010). Another danger here is when researchers suggest that coherent narratives are related to good mental health but this can then be experienced as pathologizing by those service users who hear voices or who have dissociative experiences.

Service User Involvement

One of the striking things for us in editing the book was that, although some promising moves are being made in involving service users and although there is much promise, there is still a long way to go. Apart from qualitative research conducted by freelance service user researchers such as Alison Faulkner and groups such as SURE, often commissioned by mental health charities rather than the NHS, there is still little involvement. Moreover, the qualitative methods used in these contexts tend to be more generic and realist in nature (although see Armes, 2009). In part, this may reflect the different agendas of service users and researchers (Thornicroft *et al.*, 2002). Researchers may be more interested in theoretical and methodological development whereas service user researchers may be more pragmatic, focused on making changes in services. Sweeney *et al.* (2009) and Wallcraft *et al.* (2009) demonstrate the range of topics addressed, methods used and challenges faced by survivor researchers.

What can be done to increase collaborative work between mental health service users and survivor researchers on the one hand and other mental health researchers (including trainees) on the other? One thing that could be done is for qualitative researchers to make contact with service user groups and to follow the models of collaborative work developed in mental health charities and some innovative NHS services. Service users could be invited to join the editorial boards of more journals and be invited to sit on the panels that evaluate research grant proposals.

One thing that strikes us is that training programmes for social workers, psychiatrists, nurses, occupational therapists, family therapists, psychotherapists and clinical psychologists are a huge and largely untapped resource for such collaborative research. Many service user groups lack serious ongoing funding and continually have to provide evidence of good outcomes to their funders. Perhaps training programmes could develop more ongoing links with such groups to provide a research resource. As a collaborative relationship develops, students and practitioners can learn important and transferable skills in how to carry out collaboration well. Many programmes require their students to conduct service evaluations and so this would make a very good fit with the needs of such community groups which could benefit from this resource and be encouraged to commission needs assessments and evaluations. However, in addition, there might also be scope for the more theoretically rich investigations sought for doctoral level dissertations. Of course, there are a number of challenges which would need to be explored at the start of such a project concerning timing and ownership. Moreover, we would not wish to encourage a colonization of the voluntary sector by professional groups. However, with time and goodwill these are usually resolvable and there are a number of models available as noted in Alison Faulkner's chapter. Pembroke and Hadfield (2010) have provided an informative and lively account of how a UK clinical psychology programme facilitated a collaborative research project between a trainee clinical psychologist and a mental health survivor.

Given the relative absence of involvement in qualitative research by service users, perhaps there is a need to draw on approaches like Participatory Action Research (PAR; Brydon-Miller & Tolman, 1997) where collaboration is built into the research process. Very little information is available on the kinds of qualitative research conducted by practitioners on training programmes. In a study of clinical psychology training, Harper (in press) has noted the relative lack of research using methods like action research and, indeed, there is no chapter on PAR in this book. However, as Chapter 12 by Michael Murray and Sally Sargeant indicates, community action can be developed from a range of approaches including narrative research. *Storying Sheffield* is another innovative project. Hosted by the University of Sheffield, it involved students and people from socially excluded groups like mental health service users. They used a variety of art forms to represent life in Sheffield (www.storyingsheffield.com).

Qualitative Research and Evidence-Based Practice

The rise of qualitative research in mental health and psychotherapy over the last 10–15 years has occurred at the same time as the evidence-based practice movement has become more established. Rachel Shaw, in Chapter 2, notes that qualitative research has much to offer even systematic reviews. However, the movement is essentially based on a direct realist epistemological framework. The hierarchy of evidence, drawn from the Cochrane collaboration has five levels and qualitative research methods would really only apply to types IV (at least one well-designed observational study) and V (expert opinion, including the opinion of service users and carers; Department of Health, 1999, p. 6). It seems a little odd to outline a hierarchy of evidence without, at the same time, linking this with the kinds of questions that different methods can address. Thus, whilst randomized controlled trials are appropriate in making judgements in relation to the efficacy of interventions where the human relationship is not considered a key factor, like pharmaceuticals (although this often underestimates the power of the placebo effect; Goldacre, 2009) – they are often problematic in relation to the psychotherapies. This is not a case of special pleading – it is simply the fact that it is impossible to blind a therapist to whether they are involved in conducting psychotherapy.

Qualitative methods are much more appropriate for many of the questions professionals and service users ask. Indeed, some clinicians such as Roy-Chowdhury (2003) have argued that qualitative research can provide 'evidence' in relation to particular research questions. However, it will require an ongoing process of education, institutional legitimation and cultural change before qualitative methods and the questions they can address have parity with quantitative methods (Harper, 2008). Of course, one of the contributions that qualitative research can make to policy debates is to help rethink the assumptive framework on which policy is based.

Dissemination

Practitioners are often encouraged to 'disseminate, disseminate, disseminate'. However, often this is through fairly traditional means, usually a peer-reviewed journal, and we know that these are read by small numbers of academic researchers whereas practising clinicians are much more likely to read professional magazines and newsletters. Indeed, publication rates even through traditional means are not as high as they could be (Cooper & Turpin, 2007). We would like to see more dissemination of better quality research through these means but also through less traditional outlets. Service users, relatives and the general public are much more likely to obtain their information from the TV, Internet, radio, newspapers and magazines. Given that participants have given up their time we, as researchers, have an ethical obligation to feedback to them (if they are interested) and to a range of other stakeholders. For other researchers, peer-reviewed journals are a useful outlet whereas, for practising clinicians, books, professional newsletters, magazines and journals may be more effective. For service users and relatives there are a range of possibilities: through magazines like *Open Mind* (the charity Mind's publication) and *Asylum* (http://www.pccs-books.co.uk/section.php?xSec=280&xPage=1) or websites like the hearing voices movement's Intervoice site (www.intervoiceonline.org). Websites like www.healthtalkonline.org show that alternative forms of media are available for dissemination. Researchers can also develop links with interested and informed journalists.

As indicated in Chapter 12, there are some very innovative methods of dissemination. Barbara Schneider and colleagues disseminated their findings on housing and mental health by involving their participants in performances and film and used these stories in graphic novels (http://callhome.ucalgary.ca/performances/index.html). Similarly, the Ontario Breast Cancer Community Research Initiative at the Centre for Research in Women's Health performed focus group extracts about women's experiences with breast cancer (Gray & Sinding, 2002).

Future Directions

In the future we think there is likely to be further innovation in data collection, the use of mixed methods and triangulation of sources of data (although this is a complex area as we saw in Chapter 7). Obviously, it has not been possible to include all methods of data collection and analysis in this book. Two areas that have recently engaged qualitative researchers within British social psychology include the use of visual methods (e.g., Reavey, 2011) and methods that attempt to address issues of embodied subjectivity – for example, that the experience of emotion is an intensely physical as well as mental one (e.g., Gillies *et al.*, 2004).

We also think that there could be much more development of data collection, drawing on psychotherapeutic insights. Even when researchers use interviews, there is no reason why a single interview should suffice – important phenomenological material can be gathered over a number of interviews with the same participant. Indeed, Dallos and Smith (2008) have argued that qualitative methods could be useful in re-invigorating the case study tradition in mental health research. We would like to see much more collaboration between practitioners, researchers and service users with more service user-led and user-commissioned research. As qualitative research within mental health matures we would hope to see a greater consideration of issues of reflexivity and of issues of diversity and cultural sensitivity.

References

Armes, D.G. (2009). Mission informed discursive tactics of British Mental Health Service-User/Survivor Movement (BSUSM) resistance to formalization pressures accompanying contractual relationships with purchasing authorities. *Journal of Mental Health, 18,* 344–352.

Brydon-Miller, M. & Tolman, D.L. (Eds.) (1997). Transforming psychology: Interpretive and participatory research methods (special issue). *Journal of Social Issues, 53* (4).

Cooper, M. & Turpin, G. (2007). Clinical psychology trainees' research productivity and publications: An initial survey and contributing factors. *Clinical Psychology and Psychotherapy, 14*, 54–62.

Dallos, R. & Smith, J.A. (2008). Practice as research and research as practice: How the qualitative case study can invigorate clinical psychology. *Clinical Psychology Forum, 182*, 18–22.

Department of Health. (1999). *National service framework for mental health.* London: Department of Health.

Gergen, K.J. (1994). Mind, text, and society: Self-memory in social context. In U. Neisser & R. Fivush (Eds.) *The remembering self: Construction and accuracy in the self-narrative* (pp. 78–104). Cambridge: Cambridge University Press.

Gillies, V., Harden, A., Johnson, K., Reavey, P., Strange, V. & Willig, C. (2004). Women's collective constructions of embodied practices through memory work: Cartesian dualism in memories of sweating and pain. *British Journal of Social Psychology, 43*, 99–112.

Goldacre, B. (2009). *Bad science.* London: Fourth Estate.

Gray, R. & Sinding, C. (2002). *Standing ovation: Performing social science research about cancer.* Lanham, MD: AltaMira Press.

Harper, D. (2003). Developing a critically reflexive position using discourse analysis. In L. Finlay & B. Gough (Eds.) *Reflexivity: A practical guide for researchers in health and social sciences* (pp. 78–92). Oxford: Blackwell Science.

Harper, D. (2008). Clinical psychology. In C. Willig & W. Stainton Rogers (Eds.) *Handbook of qualitative research in psychology* (pp. 430–454). London: Sage.

Harper, D. (in press). Surveying qualitative research teaching on British clinical psychology training programmes 1992–2006: A changing relationship? *Qualitative Research in Psychology.*

Herlihy, J., Scragg, P. & Turner, S. (2002). Discrepancies in autobiographical memories: Implications for the assessment of asylum seekers: repeated interviews study. *British Medical Journal, 324*, 324–327.

Hyvärinen, M., Hydén, L.C., Saarenheimo, M. & Tamboukou, M. (Eds.) (2010). *Beyond narrative coherence.* Amsterdam: John Benjamins.

Parker, I. (2005). *Qualitative psychology: Introducing radical research.* Maidenhead: Open University Press.

Pembroke, L. & Hadfield, J. (2010). Psychological research mentored by a survivor activist: Having your cake and eating it! *Clinical Psychological Forum, 209*, 9–12.

Reavey, P. (2011). *Visual psychologies: Using and interpreting images in qualitative research.* London: Routledge.

Roy-Chowdhury, S. (2003). Knowing the unknowable: What constitutes evidence in family therapy? *Journal of Family Therapy, 25*, 64–85.

Salway, S., Allmark, P., Barley, R., Higginbottom, G., Gerrish, K. & Ellison, G.T.H. (2009). Social research for a multiethnic population: Do the research ethics and standards guidelines of UK Learned Societies address this challenge? *21st Century Society, 4*, 53–81.

Shackman, J. (1985). *A handbook on working with, employing and training interpreters.* Cambridge: National Extension College.

Smith, J.A. (2004). Reflecting on the development of interpretative phenomenological analysis and its contribution to qualitative research in psychology. *Qualitative Research in Psychology, 1*, 39–54.

Sweeney, A., Beresford, P., Faulkner, A., Nettle, M. & Rose D. (Eds.) (2009). *This is survivor research.* Ross-on-Wye: PCCS Books.

Thornicroft, G., Rose, D., Huxley, P., Dale, G. & Wykes, T. (2002). What are the research priorities of mental health service users? *Journal of Mental Health, 11,* 1–5.

Tribe, R. & Raval, H. (2003). Working with interpreters in mental health. Hove: Brunner-Routledge.

Vara, R. & Patel, N. (in press). Working with interpreters in qualitative psychological research: Methodological and ethical issues. *Qualitative Research in Psychology.*

Wallcraft, J., Schrank, B. & Amering, M. (Eds.) (2009). *Handbook of service user involvement in mental health research.* Chichester: Wiley-Blackwell.

Index

Qualitative Research Methods in Mental Health and Psychotherapy: A Guide for Students and Practitioners, First Edition.
Edited by D. Harper and A.R. Thompson.
© 2012 John Wiley & Sons, Ltd. Published 2012 by John Wiley & Sons, Ltd.

Printed and bound by CPI Group (UK) Ltd, Croydon, CR0 4YY

27/10/2024

14580292-0005